THERAPEUTIC OPTIONS FOR ASDs

Therapeutic Options for ASDs

G. Hema Gowri

KANISHKA PUBLISHERS, DISTRIBUTORS
NEW DELHI-110 002

KANISHKA PUBLISHERS, DISTRIBUTORS
4697/5-21 A, Ansari Road, Daryaganj
New Delhi-110 002
Phones : 2327 0497, 2328 8285
Fax : 011-2328 8285
E-mail: kanishka_publishing@yahoo.co.in

Therapeutic Options for ASDs
First Published 2010

ISBN 978-81-8457-223-0

PRINTED IN INDIA

Published by Madan Sachdeva for Kanishka Publishers, Distributors, 4697/5-21A, Ansari Road, Daryaganj, New Delhi-110 002, Typeset by Sunshine Graphics, Delhi, and Printed at Rajdhani Printers, Delhi.

Preface

The opportunity to write this book has been an important watershed in my professional development. It reflects what I have learned and what I have been taught by the committed professionals, Individuals with Autism Spectrum Disorders and their families with whom I have interacted over the past fourteen years.

Our knowledge about ASD is increasing on a regular basis and the Therapies being used are also changing accordingly. The fruit of past research in ASD includes myriad interventions, approaches, and techniques. Exploring and deciding which approach or method is suitable to this heterogenic group is a biggest challenge for the family, professionals, therapists or trainees. The effort to provide the appropriate and relevant material in Therapeutic area in a brief text-form is a motivating challenge for me. My experience with the parents/family members/special educators/trainees whoever residing in remote part our country made me to present simplified overview of this topic.

Indeed, it is a difficult task to present all the basic essential aspects into a limited number of chapter and pages of a brief text. However the attempt is being made to present what is essential both from the angle and scope of the subject as well as the needs and demands. Throughout the text, I have tried to make the topics readable and stimulating as possible. The topics planned by RCI experts for DSE (ASD) is a gifted shortcut for me in preparing this manual. My heartfelt gratitude to RCI's team and I oblige to RCI forever.

A major ongoing influence in my own growth as a professional in special education field is Prof. P. Jeya Chandran who often offers encouragement and opportunities to become competent. He motivated me to develop the confidence to extend my understanding and skills as a special educator. He remains as the backbone support and deserves all my credible due to him.

I want to give special acknowledgement to Ms. Merry Barua who has been particularly instrumental, inspiring role model and main pillar in implementing knowledge in the field of ASDs. My sincere thanks are due to her.

My special thanks to Ms. Indu Chaswal and Ms. Reena Bhattachary for their encouragement and facilitation to widen and share my knowledge in preparing this manual. Many other friends and colleagues, who as unmentioned, were also influential, supportive and highly appreciated. I hope they will know that they were remembered as well.

I absolutely want to thank my family members especially my parents whom often given freedom to explore and fulfill my dreams in the field of special education. My big salute to my beloved parents.

The last but not the least I express deep sense of gratitude everyone associated with this manual.

I hope this manual will prove its worth and be of benefit to all those for whom it has been specially tailored. Any suggestion for its improvement will be gratefully accepted and appreciated. The suggestions will help us to add it in the revised version of this manual.

G. Hema Gowri

Contents

1

Introduction

I. INTERVENTION FOR AUTISM: THE EVOLUTION OF APPROACH

The study of Autism is relatively new. A review of fairy tales, myths and old medical records indicates that throughout history there have been people with autism. Superstitions were developed to explain the unexpected and the unusual individual with such distinctive features seemed to be 'possessed' by devils or sometimes by angles. They were often referred as idiots, witches, wild people, fools and sometimes prophets.

The condition received little attention until Leo Kanner (1943) described the syndrome that he called early infantile autism. Although Kanner viewed infantile autism as distinct from childhood schizophrenia he concluded that when children with autism grew up they were likely to develop schizophrenia.

Following the year, Hans Asperger (1944) described as Autistic Psychopathy in childhood. Once Kanner and Asperger gave Autism an identity within the medical community, theories abounded as to the causes of Autism and appropriate care for person with autism.

Autistic spectrum disorders is a recently adapted phrase. Many of early theories and associated treatments of autism have been reputed. The knowledge base and understanding of autism continues to expand as research progresses, there is yet much to learn. Even the diagnostic criteria and labels have changed over the years. Each of the four revisions of the DSM reflects the knowledge base at the time of publication and uses different terminology. Autism is a very complex disorder with a short history of documentation.

Autism, for most of the half century that label has been in use, many have understood it as a life sentence for the individuals to whom it has been applied. Most were expected to have serious and permanent deficits in communication, play, relating to others, and learning. A very small proportion of people with autism (less than 5%) might be expected to achieve independent functioning as adults, but even within the tiny group many retain at least some autistic characteristic.

Historically, most people with autism spectrum disorder (ASD) have required extensive treatment and supports throughout their lives. Today the mainstream position is that ASD is a "severely incapacitating lifelong developmental disability." It is considered treatable; indeed a vide variety of treatments, therapies and techniques are claimed to help people with ASD, and new ones are invented regularly.

A brief review of prevailing ideas about causes of autism and its treatment:

Historical Perspective on Prevailing Ideas about Causes of Autism and its Treatment

Pre-1960s

- Autism thought to be psychodynamic *i.e.* caused by the mother's emotional coldness
- Autism poorly defined—little or no differentiation
- Few specialist approaches
- Autism regarded as a variant of schizophrenia

Post-1960s

- Psychodynamic theory debunked
- Specialist education pioneered
- Autism variously attributed to
    - Biomedical factors *e.g.* GI or allergies
    - Environmental factors *e.g.* toxins
    - Vaccines
    - Genetic factors
    - Predisposition
- Functional neuro developmental factors

1970s

- Growth of interest in biomedical treatments
- Specialist 'autism specific' education established
- Growth in use of behavioural treatments
- Growth in use of drugs

1980s

- Growing sophistication of behavioural treatments
- Interest in autism specific approaches *e.g.* TEACCH imported from USA
- Emergence of alternative approaches
- More drugs

1990s

- Resurgence of interest in biomedical treatments
- Generic application of structured autism specific approaches (*e.g.* growth of TEACCH)
- Changes in way autism diagnosed
- Growth of cognitive behavioural approaches
- More drugs

Current Situation

- Renewed interest in biomedical explanations and treatments
- Behavioural interventions (ABA) remain popular
- No shortage of new approaches—compelling anecdotal evidence—mostly unsupported.
- No drug for autism—but some medications for secondary effects or co-morbidities may be useful
- Growing application of cognitive behavioural approaches

Introduction to Intervention in ASD

An intervention is any action – such as treatment, a therapy, or the provisions of a service – which is designed to help people with

ASDs. There are already more than 100 different interventions designed to help people with autistic spectrum disorders.

What are Interventions Supposed to do?

Different people make different claims for different intervention. But, in general, most interventions are designed to do one or more of the following:

- Cure autism
- Increase adaptive behaviours, such as social skills, communication skills or imaginative behaviours
- Reduce or eliminate problematic behaviours, such as self-harm or aggression towards others
- Treat co-existing conditions, such as epilepsy or gastro-intestinal problems
- Improve or enhance the quality of life of the person with autism

Of course, some people claim that some interventions can do all of these things.

Which Intervention Actually Work?

Most interventions appears to produce benefits of some kind, otherwise people would not use them. Unfortunately in some cases these apparent benefits are short-term, insignificant or illusory. And any benefits may be outweighed by the financial and emotional costs of the intervention, or the dangers inherent in some therapies.

At present there is very little scientifically valid research into the effectiveness of most autism interventions. However, we do know that some interventions are more promising than others.

For example, there is strong evidence to support the effectiveness of interventions such as early intensive behavioural intervention for young children. And there is equally strong scientific evidence to show that some interventions, such as facilitated communication are not effective.

Having said all that, each person with autism is different and what works for one person may not work for another.

It is very difficult to evaluate intervention due to various reasons such as—

- It can be difficult and time consuming to set up properly controlled scientific studies.
- The researchers may have commercial interests in proving the success of intervention
- What works for one person with autism may not work for another.
- An individual's symptoms may 'spontaneously' improve over time, irrespective of which intervention is used.
- The realities of family life may interfere with the research.
- The people involved in the trial of an intervention may really, really want it to work. So much so that they see significant improvements where there are none.

The number of interventions – therapeutic approaches, philosophies, treatments, individual therapies and services, used in ASDs are increasing. Many of these will make claims for effectiveness in excess of what is supported by the available research evidence.

Many interventions are well-established, others are quite new. Some may fall out of favour, sometimes later returning in rebranded form. Some will have impressive credentials with extravagant claims based on anecdotal reports or incomplete science. However, unless caused by a specific known medical conditions such as PKU (phenylketonuria) there is no compelling evidence to link any particular intervention or approach with prevention or 'cure' or 'recovery' of autism. The core features of autism have been shown to be resistant to intervention by whatever means, although significant improvement have been noted. People with autism may share a number of similar behavioural and other characteristics but each one is unique. Approaches must be sensitive to their uniqueness and to their individuality.

Evolution of Approaches Moved from Myths to Reality

There are many common myths that surround autism. Here we try to separate fact from fiction.

Myth	*Reality*
Autism (including Asperger syndrome) is a rare condition	Autism is no longer seen as a rare condition
Autism is a new phenomenon	The first detailed description of a child we now know had autism was written in 1799 by Jean Itard in his account of the wild boy of Aveyron.
Autism is the result of emotional deprivation or emotional stress	Autism is a complex developmental disability involving a biological or organic defect in the functioning of the brain
Autism is due to parental rejection or cold, unemotional parents	Autism has nothing whatsoever to do with the way parents bring up their children
A person with autism cannot be educated	With the right structured support within and outside of school, individuals with autism can be helped to reach their full potential
People with autism wish to avoid social contact	People with autism are often keen to make friends but, due to their disability, find this difficult
People with autism look different from other people	Autism is an invisible disability—most people with an autism spectrum disorder look just like anyone else who does not have this condition
Autism is a childhood condition	Autism is a lifelong developmental disability with no cure. Children with autism grow up to be adults with autism
All people with autism have a extraordinary ability like the Dustin Hoffman character in the film *Rainman*	People with autism who have an extraordinary talent are referred to as 'autistic savants'. Savants are rare: Savant ability is more frequently associated with those having some form of autism rather than with other disabilities. Current thinking holds that at most 1 or 2 in 200 individuals with an autism spectrum disorder might have a genuine savant talent. However, there is no reliable frequency estimate as yet as there is still no register of people with autism in the UK.

II. THE RANGE OF INTERVENTIONS: FACTS AND FICTION

No development disorders has thrown up diverse a range of treatments as has ASDs. No single treatment is best, and treatment is typically tailored to the child's need. Treatments fall into two major categories: Educational Intervention and Medical Management.

Studies of intervention have methodological problems that prevent definitive conclusions about efficacy. Although many psycho-social interventions have some positive evidence, suggesting that some form of treatment is preferable to no treatment, the methodological quality of systematic revenues of these studies has generally been poor. Intensive, sustained special education programmes and behaviour therapy early in life can help children with ASD acquire self-care, social, and job skills and often can improve functioning and decrease symptom severity and maladaptive behaviours, claims that intervention by around age three years as crucial are not substantiated. Available approaches include ABA, developmental models, structured teaching, speech and language therapy, social skills therapy and occupational therapy. The limited research on the effectiveness of adult residential programmes shows mixed results.

Many medications are used to treat problems associated with ASD. More than half children are prescribed psycho-active drugs or anti-convulsants with the most common drug classes being anti-depressants, stimulants, and anti-psychotics. Aside from anti-psychotics, there is scant reliable research about the effectiveness or safely of drug treatments for adolescents and adults with ASD.

Many alternative therapies and intervention are available, ranging from elimination of diet to chelation therapy. Few are supported by scientific study.

III. APPROACHES TO INTERVENTION : MEDICAL, BEHAVIOURAL, COMMUNICATION AND OTHERS

Approaches differ however, in their theoretical basis and consequent intervention paradigms, with a range including providing a structured education setting, behavioural approaches which shape and modify behaviours, medical approaches, communication approaches, sensory motor approach etc.

A. Medical Intervention

Medical methods do not cure, control or change the core problems/ deficits in any significant way. Treatment is generally targeted at symptom clusters and treatment can also be beneficial for the complications or associated disorder. Physicians are in the unique position of being an objective voice that families will respond to. The medical professional makes a very important contribution to the well-being outcome of children with ASDs and their families.

Medical Issues/Medications

- *Autism Spectrum Medical Issues*: A family's personal journey in dealing with the treatment of Autism.
- *Allergies and Food Sensitivities*: People with autism are more susceptible to allergies and food sensitivities than the average person; and this is likely due to their impaired immune system. A brief discussion of allergies and food sensitivities are given below.
- *Vitamin B6 and Magnesium*: An effective intervention for many autistic children and adults is the use of vitamin B6 (pyridoxine) and magnesium. For over 30 years, parents have given B6 and magnesium to their children and have observed benefits ranging from mild to dramatic. B6 and magnesium are safe and inexpensive.
- *Evaluating the Effects of Medication*: When a medication is being evaluated to modify the behaviour of a person with autism, one must assess the risks versus the benefits. The benefits of the medication must outweigh the risks. Some medications can damage the nervous system and other internal organs, such as the liver.
- *Vaccines and Autism Theory*: Current scientific evidence does not support the hypothesis that measles-mumps-rubella (MMR) vaccine, or any combination of vaccines, causes the development of autism, including regressive forms of autism.
- *Autism from Mercury Poisoning*: Thimerosal is an organic compound that contains mercury, or an 'organomercurial' and can cause Mercury poisoning.
- *Autism and Element Imbalances*: Much concern has been raised over the link between exposure to heavy metal

toxins and neurological brain damage associated with learning and behavioural disorders in children. Indeed, research shows that exposure to heavy metals such as lead and mercury can impair brain development at very early ages-even at low doses previously deemed 'harmless'.

- *Autism and Amino Acids*: Clinical and anecdotal evidence suggests that diet and digestive function play important roles in influencing symptoms in many autistic children. Amino acids are the chemical building blocks of key neurotransmitters that act on the brain to influence mood and behaviour.
- *Autism and Fatty Acids*: Increasing evidence suggests that essential fatty acids, which are critical nutrients for the brain, may be especially important for children suffering from developmental disorders like autism.
- *Autism and Medical Marijuana*: Some families have found marijuana (MMJ) to be nothing short of miraculous. Some of the symptoms MMJ has ameliorated include anxiety—even severe anxiety—aggression, panic disorder, generalised rage, tantrums, property destruction and self-injurious behaviour.
- *Naltrexone and Autism*: In the past year, naltrexone has received a great deal of media attention. Although there have only been a handful of studies on the effectiveness of naltrexone, these reports are quite encouraging.
- *Biomedical and Dietary Treatments*: While there are no drugs, vitamins or special diets that can correct the underlying neurological problems that seem to cause autism, parents and professionals have found that some drugs used for other disorders are sometimes effective in treating some aspects of or behaviours associated with autism.
- Autism and secretin.
- *Treatment*: There is no standard, universally accepted treatment of autism; in fact, every single method has its detractors. General approaches may be summarised as follows.
- *Treatment of PDDNOS*: No one therapy or method will work for all individuals with Autistic Disorder or PDDNOS. Many professionals and families will use a range of treatments simultaneously, including behaviour modification,

structured educational approaches, medications, speech therapy, occupational therapy, and counselling.

- *Dietary Autism Treatment*: Autism may be aided by a gluten-free, casein-free diet.
- *Gluten Free Casein Free Diet and Autism*: Explanation of the diet, menus, sources of foods, message board.

B. Behavioural Approaches

The third element of the triad of impairments relates to the behaviour of individuals with autism. Behavioural approaches rest on the theory of Skinner (1951) that learning is development, and all behaviour is learned. Using associative learning and operant conditioning, behavioural responses can be modified by positive and negative reinforcement. This approach was developed on the theoretical basis that persons with autism had not learned the behaviours of typically developing children because they could not respond to the typical environment, and so, it was necessary for the environmental input to be altered to condition behavioural responses (Lovaas 1987). A particular behavioural approach "Applied Behavioural Analysis" is used by Lovaas and colleagues which involves breaking a skill into small steps and teaching each step a discrete trial technique. Other behavioural approaches have incorporated developments in behavioural methodology, such as 'errorless discrimination learning' and 'functional analysis'. Prizant, whetherby and Rydell (2000) draw a distinction between earlier discrete trial training (DTT) behavioural approach, and the contemporary applied behaviour analysis (CABA) approach, which involves behavioural reinforcement for appropriate responses but also uses naturalistic settings and structured minimally interactions.

ABA style intervention aim to apply scientifically validated principles of behaviour.

Some popular ABA style interventions include:

(a) *Early Intensive Behavioural Intervention (EIBI)*: EIBI methods are intended to increase behaviours (e.g. on task behaviours, social interactions) teach new skills (e.g. life skills, communication skills, or social skills), maintain existing behaviours, generalize or transfer behaviour across situations or responses, and to restrict or narrow condition under which interfering behaviours. (e.g., self injury or stereotypy).

(b) *Learning Experiences*: An alternative programme for pre-schoolers and parents (LEAP) includes behavioural skill-training programme for parents.

(c) *Pivotal Response Training (PRT)*: PRT is a behavioural treatment intervention. It is a naturalistic intervention developed by Robert L. Koegel. PRT aims to increase the generalization of new skills by increasing motivation, including components such as child choice, turn-taking, reinforcing attempts and interspersing maintenance tasks.

(d) *Positive Behaviour Supports (PBS)*: The PBS process involves engineering the environment to prevent problems from occuring: teaching individually acceptable alternative behaviours to replace problem behaviours; and consistently providing for positive consequences that encourage appropriate behaviour outcomes over time.

(e) *Pyramid Approach*: Includes using Picture Exchange Communication (PECS): The application of ABA methods to teach PECS is the intervention.

(f) *Hansen Programme/More Than Words (MTW)*: Integrates more traditional behavioural approaches with developmental, socio-pragmatic approaches into a single programme.

(g) *Natural Environment Training, Naturalistic Learning*: This method generally is used in conjunction with DTT-ABA and uses child's immediate interest and activities as a reward.

Individual curricula and teaching approaches based on behavioural approaches may vary but commonly used approaches are Applied Behavioural Analysis (ABA), Discrete Trial Training (DTT) Applied Virtial Behaviour (AVB) and Lovaas method.

Some elements of behavioural approaches are included in other approaches such as Division TEACCH; but TEACCH would not use behavioural approaches in developing interpersonal understanding, considering them to be unsuited to promoting this type of development.

C. Communication Approach

Communication is one of the most well-researched in ASD. Communication is a core difficulty for all children with ASD, but there is a wide diversity of skills among individuals. Impairments can range from a failure to develop any functional communication at all to the development of apparently good language, but with unusual elements. Communication is a complex process and has several different aspects.

1. Receptive communication
2. Expressive communication
3. Joint attention
4. Symbol use
5. Social pragmatic skills
6. Echolalia
7. Unconventional behaviour

Communication Interventions

The AZ Method: The AZ method uses video to develop language skills in people with ASD. The video technique illustrates everyday objects and uses voice-over to identify each. Each video stresses different things, including concepts. Life skills and facial expressions used to describe emotions are also taught through the use of videos.

Facilitated Communication: Facilitated Communication is a technique by which a trained professional, a facilitator, supports the hand, arm or shoulder of an individual with communication impairments so that the person with the impairment can either point to or press the keys of a communication device. If successful, the individual who was previously unable to communicate can do so through typing or spelling out words.

Neuro-Linguistic Programming: Neuro-Linguistic Programming is the relationship between neurology, linguistics and observable patterns of behaviour, to help build self confidence and capability.

Picture Exchange Communication System: The Picture Exchange Communication System (PECS) is an augmentative communication training package that allows children and adults with ASD, who comprehend relate to pictures, to initiate communication.

Picture Rehearsal: Picture rehearsal is an instructional strategy that uses repeated practice of a sequence of behaviours by presenting the sequence to the individual in the form of pictures and accompanying script.

Signed Speech or Simultaneous Communication: Teaching sign language and speech at the same time is often referred to as Signed

Speech or Simultaneous Communication. Although this form of communication is not universally understood and used by others, it is one form of communication that may be considered when teaching communication to persons with ASD.

Speech/Language Therapy: Speech/language therapy is a service provided when a person's speech or language is markedly different from that of others of the same age, sex, or ethnic group; when a person's speech or language is difficult to understand; when a person is overly concerned about his or her own speech; or when a person frequently avoids communicating with others. Difficulties may involve articulation, voice, stuttering or language, including semantics, syntax and pragmatics. Although individuals with ASD may evidence a variety of speech and language difficulties, their primary deficit appears to be in the area of pragmatics or social communication.

D. Sensory and Motor Approaches

It is recognised that people with autism can have sensory and perceptual sensitivities, unusual motor behaviours and altered sensory processing abilities (*e.g.* Bogdashina, 2003). Baranek (2002) presents a review of the efficacy of sensory and motor interventions for children with autism. She reviews studies across a range of interventions including visual therapies, Sensory Integration Therapies, sensory stimulation techniques, Auditory Integration Training (AIT), sensorimotor handling techniques, and concludes that the evidence is either inadequate or does not indicate effectiveness for such sensory and motor interventions. In one study (Mudford *et al.*, 2000) of auditory integration training the results for the control group were better than for the intervention group.

Sinha, Silove, Wheeler and Williams (2004) examined evidence for the effectiveness of AIT or other methods of sound therapy in individuals with ASD. They found that no trials assessing sound therapies other than AIT met their criteria, and that these trials still contained methodological shortcomings. Of these, three trials did not demonstrate benefits of AIT over control conditions, and three did report improvement using an outcome measurement the validity of which the authors question. They conclude that more research is needed in this area.

The Higashi 'Daily Life Therapy' approach (Kitahara, 1983) emphasises strenuous exercise programmes as part of a holistic approach. This approach has not has systematic evaluation.

Sensory-Motor Interventions

Auditory Training

Berard Method: Developed by Dr. Guy Berard, this method was designed to assist people with auditory processing problems.

Tomatis Method: Developed by Dr. Alfred A. Tomatis, this method was the first auditory training method designed to re-educate the way we listen, communicate, and use language.

Auditory Tutorial Programmes

Earobics: This tutorial programme contains six games that are designed to teach a variety of auditory and phonological skills to children between the ages of 4 and 7 years. Older children with developmental disabilities may also benefit.

Fast ForWord: Fast ForWord uses seven games which are designed to train the brain to process sounds more efficiently and rapidly. Through this programme the length of speech sounds is altered so that the person can more easily recognise the sounds.

Dolphin Therapy: Several educational facilities have been developed which use dolphins as a therapeutic tool for persons with autism. The multi-sensory stimulation which occurs in the dolphin environment may allow for increased communication, social, and sensory improvements as well as boosting immune systems for persons with ASD.

Exercise: Other than the obvious benefits of exercise, several research studies have shown that vigorous or strenuous exercise is often associated with decreases in self-stimulatory behaviours, hyperactivity, aggression, self-injury, and destructiveness. Exercise through school or community programmes is helpful as well as through the development of an individual exercise programme.

Higashi (Daily Life Therapy)

This technique was pioneered by Dr. Kiyo Kitawa at the Higashi School in Japan and provides education and emphasizes greatly vigorous physical education and the arts. For more information on internet, contact the Boston Higashi School.

Hippotherapy (Therapeutic Horseback Riding)

The benefits of therapeutic horseback riding for persons with ASD are many. Therapy builds upon the psycho-social benefits of riding a horse, and adds improvements in physical components as well. The motion and heat of the horse not only aid a rider's blood circulation and reflexes, but also gently exercise the rider's spinal column, providing a combination of sensory and neurological input that can be used to address a variety of disabilities, including ASD.

Irlen Lenses and Scotopic Sensitivity

Scotopic sensitivity/irlen syndrome is a visual-perceptual problem which occurs in some people with learning/reading disorders, ASD, and other developmental disorders.

Helen Irlen has developed two methods to treat Scotopic Sensitivity: (1) the use of coloured transparencies or overlays to improve reading; and (2) tinted glasses to improve one's visual perception of his/her environment.

Occupational Therapy

Occupational therapy is the therapeutic use of self-care, work, and play activities to increase independent function, enhance development, and prevent disability. It may include adaptation of task or environment to achieve maximum independence and to enhance quality of life. For ASD, an occupational therapist may use a variety of strategies: sensory integration addressing developmental, gross and fine motor needs; visual structuring; movement therapy to address motor needs; listening therapy; and provide combination therapy with speech/language pathologists.

Self-Management

Self-management refers to the individual achieving personal autonomy. The goal for the person with ASD is to shift super-vision and control from a parent, caregiver, job coach, or employer to the person himself/herself.

Sensory Integration Therapy

Sensory integration theory was developed by A. Jean Ayres, Ph.D., OTR/L. Sensory integration refers to the organization of our senses to give us an understanding of ourselves and what is going on in the world around us. Our perceptions of taste, touch, smell, hearing, vision, balance, movement, body awareness, etc., are combined and organised by our brain to give us a clear 'picture'. Each of our different senses provides us with a piece of the puzzle that combines to form a picture.

Alert Programme

The alert programme helps children learn a repertoire of strategies that strengthens their abilities to learn, interact with others, and work or play. Children not only learn to monitor their alertness, but to improve in self-esteem and self-confidence skills. This programme was developed by occupational therapists Mary Sue Williams and Sherry Shellenberger.

Brushing Programme

The brushing programme was developed by Pat Wilbarger, an occupational therapist, who believes that brushing provides assistance with sensory defensiveness.

Sensory Diet

This concept is based on the idea that each individual requires a certain amount of activity and sensation to be alert, adaptable, and skilful. Some persons who are sensory defensive (see Brushing Programme) respond well to a sensory diet, which means that a variety of different activities are used to reduce sensory defensiveness. Activities may include deep pressure, specific movement, neutral warmth, activities in upside down postures, joint traction and compression, heal to head rocking, activities requiring heavy work to muscles and others.

Vision Therapy/Training

Vision therapy is a process of retraining the visual perceptual system so that it functions with optimal efficiency. The process follows a sequence of steps aimed at improving the visual system.

E. Appraisal of Approaches (See table on page 18)

Extent of use and effectiveness of approaches to teaching children with ASD will be organised in relation to

(*i*) Understood casual processes and areas of impact.
(*ii*) Functional focus of the approach.
(*iii*) The personal or interpersonal focus of approach.
(*iv*) The social context of the approach.

This allows the range of approaches to be systematically presented in relation to key features of their application.

IV. UNDERSTANDING THE 'WHOLE' OF IT

There are many types of interventions available today for autistic individuals, including nutritional, biomedical, educational, sensory and behavioural. When beginning a new intervention, it is important to be as objective as possible to determine whether the treatment truly helped the person. If the treatment is not helping, then it does not make sense to continue it especially if it involves a great deal of time, money or effort.

Issues Around Effectiveness of Interventions

The intervention approaches outlines above indicate contrasts in theoretical approach – and in some cases would be mutually exclusive, and impact upon other daily events and opportunities for a child to socialise. Clearly it is important to know which interventions are effective and which would suit any particular child, in relation to individual characteristics, age and context, which would allow the child to be independent.

Evaluating an intervention approach, however, can be difficult in relation to people with autism who form a heterogeneous group. Issues arise in relation to numbers of participants in an evaluation study, comparability of individual characteristics. The ethics and recruitment of a control group, the random assignment of participant to comparative groups – all of which pose methodological difficulties for comparative intervention paradigms.

Looking closely at the methodologies involved in various studies they found that, while most approaches provided some evidence of effectiveness, they were very variable in scientific terms.

Evidence of effectiveness of approaches in supporting the teaching children with autism in more recent years needs further investigation.

Appraisal of Approach

Effectiveness and Appraisal of Approach Types in Relation to Teaching Children with Autism

Approach/Intervention Area	*Evidence of Effectiveness*	*Possible Strengths*	*Possible Drawbacks*
Structured Educational Environment	Studies tend to be uncontrolled or of confounding design, but positive outcomes are reported	Lifelong adaptations Individualised programming Visual aids and routines aid independence Reduce stress	Dependence on external structure Lack of social/group learning experience
Behavioural	Methodological difficulties with studies. Results report positive outcomes	Certain response behaviours can be trained and functioning improved	Response behaviour does not indicate understanding Not clear what component of intervention is active Time intensity may preclude involvement in other effective interventions Long-term benefits uncertain
PECS	Studies tend to be uncontrolled or with small numbers and not randomised participants	Can provide an alternative means of expressive communication and promote communicative initiating behaviour	Requires consistency and structured contexts which may be difficult to achieve and may preclude spontaneous and playful interactions.

(*Contd.*)

Approach/Intervention Area	*Evidence of Effectiveness*	*Possible Strengths*	*Possible Drawbacks*
Developmental/Interactive Approaches	Studies tend to be uncontrolled or with small numbers and not randomised participants Very positive results reported	Directly address child's motivation to engage and be involved socially Developing self and relationships Can promote symbolic and imaginative abilities Parents can use spontaneous opportunities Based on fundamental processes of typical development Does not have to be time intensive	May involve a lack of structure May need targetted goals
Music Therapy	Studies tend to be uncontrolled or with small numbers and not randomised participants Positive results reported	Can encourage interpersonal connectedness and processes of communication without speech or content	Not always shared regulation of activity
Parental Programmes	Limited forms of evaluative evidence Positive perceptions reported	Informing and empowering parents	May be time limited
Peer Mediated Interventions	Studies tend to be uncontrolled or with small numbers and not randomised participants Positive results reported	Addressing social integration Can aid generalization of abilities Can promote friendships Can promote symbolic and imaginative abilities	Peers may require training Peer input may vary

(*Contd.*)

Approach/Intervention Area	*Evidence of Effectiveness*	*Possible Strengths*	*Possible Drawbacks*
Social Interaction Groups	Studies tend to be uncontrolled or with small numbers and not randomised participants Positive results reported	Can increase socio-emotional understanding, social competence communication and friendships can aid generalization of abiliaties	Need to avoid teaching 'splinter skills' in isolation
Socio-Constructive/Cognitive Approaches	Studies tend to be uncontrolled or with small numbers and not randomised participants Positive results reported	Can help with problem solving, emotional understanding, understanding meanings and social interaction. Can teach about feelings and intentions and help to guide behaviour Individually targetted	Requires identifying the particular cause of a difficulty in context May require many versions made of a social story
Sensory and Motor	Studies tend to be uncontrolled or with small numbers and not randomised participants Some results showed no positive effective of AIT	May improve aspects of functioning in some individuals	Can be time consuming to be effective AIT reported to have adverse the effect in certain individuals
Bio-medical	Studies tend to be uncontrolled or with small numbers and not randomised participants Mixed rusults reported	May improve aspects of functioning in some individuals	Some medications could be harmful Further research is needed

2

Medical Intervention

I. UNDERLYING RATIONALE FOR MEDICAL INTERVENTIONS

Autism Spectrum Disorder (ASD) are now recognised as neurobiologically based conditions. ASDs are similar to other neurodevelopmental disabilities, are generally not 'curable', and individuals with ASD require ongoing medical monitoring and care, as would any person with a chronic medical condition. Medical methods do not cure, control or change the core problems/ deficits in any significant way. Autism is an enormously heterogeneous disorder with a wide range of symptom expression across individuals as well as across disorders on the autism spectrum. There is also significant co-morbidity in this population, with affective and attention disorders commonly observed. All of these factor make effective pharmacological treatment a challenging proposition.

To add to the challenge, no medication is available that effectively treats the core social and communication deficits that define autism. Current drug therapy have been termed palliative treatments, and behavioural interventions remain the mainstay of treatment. As neither genetic nor environmental causes of autism have been identified, it has been difficult to firmly establish molecular mechanisms that would serve as potential targets for pharmacological intervention. Thus, medications that have been tested for efficacy in individuals with autism have been selected on the basis of their effectiveness in relevant disorders.

Medicating a person with ASD can be a catch-22 situation. These person may need medication to function better within society, but the body of an autistic person does its best to reject medication. Medical tests have shown that autistic people are more prone to drug reactions and rare side effects that doctors don't often seem to worry about. People on the spectrum are more likely to have paradoxical reactions, which occur when a drug should function one way but does the opposite. And, generally speaking, the autistic population is more likely to experience drug toxicity, or toxic effects from a drug regardless of the amount taken. An autistic person's body doesn't always get rid of medications as fast as the average person's dose. As a result, a person on the spectrum may need to start a medication at a much lower dose than normal and likely remain on that low dose.

Rational Drug Therapy for Person with ASD

- Use proper titration rate
  - Start slow, go slow
- Ensure adequate dose
  - Target: minimum effective dose
- Ensure adequate duration of medication trial
  - 2-8 weeks for neuroleptics, AEDs
  - SNRIs/SSRIs
  - If partial response, allow for longer duration of observation
- Evaluate for compliance/side effects
  - Utilise blood levels if applicable
  - Assess for typical responses
  - Monitor for side-effects
    - Physical/neurological examination
    - Laboratory testing
- Ensure proper diagnosis
  - Determine if there are co-morbid diagnosis
  - Evaluate whether proper therapeutic targets have been chosen
- Evaluate whether there is an underlying systematic trigger for the maladaptive behaviour, such as pair or underlying medical condition
- Ensure that non-pharmacological interventions are maximised
- Attempt to secure objective or quantitative outcome measures

- Avoid polypharmacy
  - If necessary, use it rationally with compatible drugs
- Periodic review of regimen
  - Consider medical reversals
    - Tapering/discontinuing medication to see if it is still exerting a benefit, while monitoring behaviour for stability or worsening.

Medications can

- Address some of the symptoms that often occur with autism (like anxiety or depression),
- Reduce some of the physical and mental causes of certain behaviours often associated with autism (like seizures, poor digestion and some sensitivities),
- Help some people with autism begin to cope with their environment.

Medications can't cure, control or change the core problems/ deficits in any significant way. There is no single best treatment package for all children with autism spectrum disorders.

II. MEDICATION AND HYPER ACTIVITY

Attention challenges in children with an ASD can be manifested in poor discrimination learning, focusing on unusual or partial ones needed for an adaptive response, and rapidly shifting attention, which may be associated with increased general activity. Some children with ASD manifest more of these hyperactive and inattentive symptoms than others. Although attention deficit hyperactivity disorder (ADHD) diagnostic criteria exclude the presence of autistic disorder, the target symptoms may sometimes respond to the same treatments as ADHD in the general population.

Clonidine, guanfaune, or imipramine may be considered in low or middle functioning child with ASD or without other neurological disorders. Naltrexone may be considered for those who do not respond to above mentioned drugs. In highly functioning individuals without other neurological disorders. Stimulants, such as methylphenidate or dextroamphetamine may be tried first. In 1995, however, Quintana *et al* described in an excellent study, that there has "a statistically significant reduction in hyperactivity without an increase in stereotypic behaviour" using methylphenidate. While 50 per cent of children with ASD are reported to respond to medication management of 'ADHD' symptoms, 20 per cent could not tolerate methylphenidate. In some kids, adverse effects are seen, including increasing irritability, paradoxical increase in hyperactivity, stereotypic behaviours, or agitation.

Significant hyperactivity can exist with autism and asperger syndrome (10-20%). The psycho-stimulants medications found positive results in ADHD + autism (2006). In higher functioning kids with ASD's response is better, more predictable and often low doses are effective. In kids with cognitive impairment (IQ<45; mental ages < 4.5) success is less likely and Idiosyncratic (negative) responses more likely, including agitation and stereotypes.

III. SPECIFIC INTERVENTION

1. Diet Therapy

Diet therapy is using diet and nutrition as therapeutic tools. When done correctly, it makes other treatments mere effective, has no side effects, and may decrease the need for drugs. The diet is not a magic cure; parents of children with autism and adults with autism have noticed that dietary interventions – such as eliminating wheat and diary products, adding supplements, or both can go so far as to reduce autistic symptoms in some people. The autistic person's digestion can improve and the diet can have positive effects on behaviour, moods and overall functioning.

A. Cleaning Up Child's Diet

A good way to clean up child's diet is to reduce junk food intake. Eliminating refined sugars and other processed foods can help improve his general well-being and improves his functioning dramatically. Avoid foods and additives such as:

- Commercial baked goods and candy
- Soft drinks and high sugar juices
- Nitrates/nitrites

- MSG (monosodium glutamate)
- Artificial colouring (such as red or blue dyes)
- Artificial sweetness (such as saccharin or aspartame)

Concentrate on whole, organically grown foods like fresh fruits and vegetables that don't contain sugars and aren't processed.

B. Gluten and Casein Free Diet (GF/CF)

There is a belief that certain food contain protein peptides that are unable to treated own in persons with ASD, causing difficulties in their brain. Some person with autism have reported mild to dramatic improvement in speech and behaviour after the removal of gluten and casein.

Gluten Containing Foods: All wheat and wheat products, rye, barley, oats.

Casein Containing Foods: All milk and milk products.

No large clinical study exists yet to back up the GF/CF diet. One school of thought says that gluten and casein are responsible for improperly broken down dietary peptides – part of the Opioid theory of autism – or that immune system dysregulation causes as abnormal immune response.

C. Other Special Red Diets

(*a*) The specific carbohydrate diet (SCD) which removes specific carbohydrates, aptly enough – is a grain-free, lactose-free and sucrose-free dietary regimn.

(*b*) Feingold's diet. Feingold's suggest that synthetic food additives can have serious learning behaviour and/or health effects on sensitive people. It advocates eliminating all additives and chemicals in the diet.

2. Allergies

Some people on the autism spectrum have high levels of the immunoglobulin IgE and multiple allergies. Many allergies are caused by food or by indoor and outdoor allergies. Food allergies usually provoke instant antibody reactions in the blood such as hives, nausea, headaches, or swelling. Nasal allergies have been shown to affect concentration and memory, two important issues for autistic children. One common allergic symptom is eczema (also known as atopic deramititis), an itchy red rash most common in the elbow creases or behind the knees.

There is difference between food allergy and food sensitivity, the terms are used interchangeably. Both can cause inflammation in your system, but food allergies provokes instant antibody reaction. Sensitivities, such as metabolic food disorders like lactose intolerance, don't affect the same part of the immune system and can be slower to act. Many children with ASD have good sensitivities.

3. Mega Vitamins

In 1995, one of the leading researchers in the field of autism, Dr. Bernard Rimland, brought together a group of exports to brainstorm the nutritional and chemical factors that might be involved in autism and PDD conditions.

Summary of DAN Protocol

DAN (Defeat Autism Now) protocol involves a combination of changes to the diet and implementation of vitamin supplement therapy as a means of producing changes in autistic behaviours. These charges include the following steps:

1. Eliminate dairy products.
2. Eliminate cereal grain products.
3. Eliminate junk foods and other food products that contain refined sugars.
4. Supplement the diet with the vitamins and mineral therapy. Below a list of the supplements and their dosages which are recommended:
    - *Calcium 300 mg Twice a Day*. This can be done in two doses or once at bed time to facilitate sleep.
    - *Magnesium*: 50 mg twice a day.
    - *Vitamin C*: 50 mg twice a day.
    - *Vitamin B5*: (Pantothenic Acid) 500 mg twice a day
    - *Vitamin B6*: 100 mg twice a day 1 multiple vitamin daily.
    - *DMG*: 50 mg twice a day.

- Pyenogenol: 50 mg twice a day.
- Gaba: 75 mg twice a day.

5. If the child is currently taking any medications especially those such as Prozac or Ritalin, it is recommended to discontinue use before beginning secretin infusions.

As with any treatment, the DAN protocol should only be undertaken with medical supervision.

Dr. Bernard Rimland has for many years championed Vitamin B6 (pyridoxine) and magnesium as effective treatments for ASD children.

Super-Nu-Thera

Since 1970, the Kirkman Company has made available megavitamin product Super-Nu-Thera, which contains the vitamins and minerals necessary for placing a child on megavitamin B6 therapy. The megavitamin formula is available both in caplets and as a ponder which may be mixed with applesauce, mashed potatoes, juices or other foods which the child finds palatable. The powder contains 500 mg of B6 per heaping teaspoon, and adequate amounts of a number of other nuitrients. Six caplets equal one heaping teaspoon of the powder determining the correct dosage is an individual matter. Super-Nu-Thera may be given together with other nutrients, such as DMG. If no improvement is seen in 30 days, it may be concluded that the child does not need the extra B6. The Super-Nu-Thera should be tapered off and stopped in that case.

Benefits of Megavitamin Therapy

The benefits which are most often observed in autistic children given B6 and the accompanying nutrients are: increased use of sounds, words or speech; improved sleeping habits; decrease in hyperactivity and irritability; better attention span; increase in interest in learning. In some cases, self-stimming, self-injurious and/ or assaultative behaviours have decreases other benefits reported have included such indications of improved health as better skin colour and complexion, and better muscle tone. Dietary supplementation is also a key ingredient of this treatment method. The combination of all the above factors have been shown to have sometimes dramatic effects on ASD, but the people at DAN are the first to admit that it is not a 'cure all' and that all improvements may not be solely the result of the protocols. Autism is a complex illness, and there are multiple factors that may influence its course.

IV. PSYCHOPHARMACOLOGY

Autism is a neurobiological disorder. Autism often has coexisting neuropsychiatric disorders, including seizure disorder, attention deficit and hyperactivity disorder (ADHD), affective disorder, anxiety disorder, obsessive-compulsive disorder, and Tourette's disorder. No etiology-based treatment modality has been developed to cure individuals with autism. Findings from preliminary studies of major neurotransmitters and other neuro-chemical agents strongly suggests that neuro-chemical factors play a major role in autism. The findings also provides the rationale for psychopharma cotherapy in person with autism.

Today, there is a consensus that autism is a neuro-biological disorder. However, no specific biological marker has been identified as the cause of autism. The specific purpose of using psychotherapeutic medications in autism is to ameliorate the psychiatric or behavioural symptoms that are interfering with the individual's ability to participate in educational, social, work, and family systems as well as to enhance the positive response to other forms of intervention in person with autism.

Intriguing research findings in the relationship between neuro-transmitters and clinical features of other neuropsychiatric disorders have led researchers to studies of major neurotransmitters and other neuro-chemical factors in autism. Although the studies are usually preliminary and often compounded by problems inherent in neuro-chemical research, the findings from the preliminary studies strongly suggest that neuro-chemical factors play a major role in ASD. The findings also provide the rationale for psycho-pharmacotherapy in individuals with ASD. A recent survey study found that about one-third of persons with autism were taking some psychotropic drug or vitamin for autism or associated behaviour or psychiatric problems.

Many investigations have reported other behavioural and/or psychiatric symptoms in persons with autism: about 60 per cent have poor attention and concentration; 40 per cent are hyperactive;

43 per cent to 88 per cent exhibit morbid or unusual pre-occupation; 37 per cent have obsessive phenomena; 16 per cent to 86 per cent show compulsion or rituals; 50 per cent to 89 per cent demonstrate stereotyped utterance; 70 per cent exhibit stereotyped mannerism; 17 per cent to 74 per cent have anxiety fears; 9 per cent to 44 per cent show depressive mood; irritability, agitation, and inappropriate affect; 11 per cent have sleep problems; 24 per cent to 43 per cent have a history of self-injury; and 8 per cent have tics. In the past, these additional symptoms were considered 'associated features' of autism. Now, more investigations argue for considering these behaviours and symptoms as features of co-existing neuro-psychiatric disorders.

Clinical Indications for Pharmacotherapy and Suggestions for Drug of Choice

The clinical symptoms in persons with autism may differ at different chronological ages. In early childhood, hyperactivity, stereotyped behaviours, irritability and temper tantrums may be prominent, whereas tic like behaviours, aggressiveness and self-injurious behaviour may characterise the child later. In adolescence and adulthood, particularly in higher-functioning individuals, depression or obsessive-compulsive phenomena may develop and interfere with functioning.

	Behavioural Problem	*Drug of Choice*
1.	Disturbance of mobility, short attention, impulsive behaviours or ADHD	Clonidine, guanfacine, or imipramine. Naltrexone may be considered for those who do not respond to earlier medicine.
2.	Resistance to change, repetitive thoughts, preservative talking, repetitive, ritualistic or compulsive behaviour, abnormal attachments, and obsessive – compulsive disorder	Clomipramine, fluoxetine, sertraline or paroxetine for children who do not have seizure disorder. For individuals with seizure clomipramine should be avoided.
3.	Stereotyped movements, or behaviours, motor and/or vocal tics or Tourette's disorder	Haloperidol or pimozide, risperidone, clonidine or fluoxetine may be tried in individuals who do not respond to haloperidol.

(*Contd.*)

	Behavioural Problem	Drug of Choice
4.	Excessive fear, worry, anxiety or generalised anxiety	Buspirone.
5.	Aggressive behaviour	Risperidone or haloperidol.
6.	Unusual sleeping patterns	Melatonin. In more severe cases imipramine, trazodone, or zolpidem may be considered.
7.	Enuresis	Imipramine and desmopressin (DDAVP).

V. SEROTONIN

Serotonin Imbalance in Autism

Neurotransmitters are powerful chemical messengers that carry messages to and from the brain. These messages are everything that you do, think, say, feel, hear, smell, touch and taste. The main neurotransmitters are serotonin, norepinephrine and dopamine. An imbalance in serotonin is believed to cause of many of the characteristic symptoms of autism. This serotonin imbalance can lead to sleep disturbances, speech delays and sensory integration problems, as serotonin regulates

- sleep
- mood
- speech
- sensory integration
- body temperature
- appetite

Selective Serotonin Reuptake Inhibitors (SSRIs)

SSRIs are anti-depressant medications used to treat a variety of conditions, including depression, anxiety and autism. It helps to keep the serotonin in the brain longer rather than being prematurely cleared out (the reuptake process).

SSRIs are commonly prescribed for children with autism, even at the age of two years old. In autism, SSRI can help dramatically with sensory integration problems, as well as problems with obsessive compulsive disorder, sleep problems and irritability. (You might see an increase in aggressive behaviours the first couple of weeks on the medication.) Currently there are six SSRIs available on the market:

- Prozac (Fluoxetine)
- Celexa (Citalopram)
- Luvox (Fluvoxamine)
- Zoloft (Sertraline)
- Paxil (Paroxetine)
- Lexapro (Escitalopram)

Regulating Serotonin Levels Using Diet

Certain foods have been found to contain high amounts of serotonin. These include: Tomatoes, bananas, plums, pecan nuts and pineapples.

By avoiding these foods, serotonin levels can be reduced. There is limited research carried out in this area.

VI. SEIZURES

Many people with autism have also have epilepsy, a disorder of the brain that results in recurrent, unprovoked seizures. Children with ASD are at increased risk for the development of seizure disorders, with 20-30 per cent or higher prevalence of epilepsy by adulthood among affected children with severe intellectual or motor disability. The seizure prevalence is less than 10 per cent among children with ASD who have less severe intellectual or motor impairments. The term antiepileptic refers to a class of drugs generally used to prevent epileptic seizures.

Common Antiepileptics

- Carbamazepine → Tegretol
- Gabapentin → Neurontin
- Lamotrigine → Lamictal
- Levetiracetam → Keppra
- Valproate → Depakote

Possible Antiepileptic Side Effects

- One of the possible severe side effects, especially with Depakote and Tegretol, is liver or bone marrow damage.
- Depakote (Valproate) also has sedative effect and can cause an upset stomach and weight gain.
- Carbamazepine has similar effect as valproate and could create a rash.
- Lamotrigine can cause severe rash. Both gabapentin and lamotrigine drugs have the same negative side effects as valproate.

Treatment with anti-convulsant medication depends on the seizure type and frequency, with close monitoring by a pediatric neurologist during medication initiation, titration and stitches.

Conclusion

Autism is an enormously heterogeneous disorder with a wide range of symptom expression across individuals as well as across disorders on the autism spectrum.

Recent autism research has discovered some valuable information about the disorder and the data can be organised into three major categories: causes, treatment and cure. The exact causes of the disorder is still unknown but some tests indicate that genetics may be responsible; some experts proposed to causative factor lives in vaccination slots, specially MMR vaccine etc. The treatment for autistic disorders has come a long way. Our understanding of the problem has grown almost as quickly as the rate of diagnosis. Hopefully, autism research will come up with mere answers to help children and adults around the world just as quickly.

Summary

Autism is an enormously heterogeneous disorder with a wide range of symptom expression across individuals as well as across disorders on the autism spectrum. To add the challenge, no medication is available that effectively treats the care social and communication deficits that deficits autism. There are a number of psychotropic medications being routinely prescribed for individuals with ASD with inadequate evidence of efficacy.

Biomedical intervention focuses on dietary change, cleaning and promoting healthy gut, promoting healthy body through natural and prescriptions medicines (vitamins and minerals), removing toxins and chemicals from the body thereby reduce inflammation, preventing and treating infections (bad germs), allergies. Medications are often used to treat behavioural problems such as aggression, self-injurious behaviours several other medications have been used to treat ASD symptoms, such as hyper activity, antidepressantants etc. A person with ASD responds atypically to medications, currently no medical treatment for the care features of autism and to cure autism.

3

Behaviour Modification Approaches

I. APPLICATION OF SKINNER'S LEARNING THEORY AND PRINCIPLES OF LEARNING TO INTERVENTION FOR VERBAL AND NON-VERBAL AND CHALLENGES IN ASD

Application of operant conditioning to education is simple and direct. In the field of special education, behaviour modification of training adaptive behaviour and eliminating maladaptive behaviour application of operant conditioning plays a large role. In modelling much of what we do? Operant conditioning has been widely applied in clinical settings (*i.e.* behaviour modification) as well as teaching (*i.e.* classroom management) and instructional development (*e.g.* programmed instruction). One of the distinctive aspects of Skinner's theory is that it is attempted to provide behavioural explanations for a broad range of cognitive phenomena. For example, Skinner explained derive (motivation) in terms of deprivation and reinforcement schedule. Skinner (1957) tried to account for verbal learning and language within the operant conditioning paradigm, although this effort was strongly rejected by linguists and psycholinguists. First Skinner defined verbal behaviour as behaviour that is reinforced through the meditation of another person's behaviour (whereas non-verbal behaviour is reinforced directly through contact with physical environment).

Operant conditioning is applied in behaviour therapy or behaviour modification programmes in teaching persons with ASD by contingently reinforcing socially adaptive behaviours and by extinguishing maladaptive behaviours.

Implications of the Theory of Operant Conditioning

Theory of operant conditioning has revolutionised the field of training or learning by bringing forward the following practical ideas and implications:

1. The learning or training process and environment must be so designed as to create minimum frustration and maximum satisfaction to learner to provide him proper reinforcement for the desired training or learning.
2. The principle of operant conditioning may be successfully applied in the task of behaviour modification.
3. The theory of operant conditioning does not attribute motivation to internal processes within the organism. It takes for granted the consequences of a behaviour or response as a source of motivation to further occurrence of that behaviour.
4. Operant conditioning lays stress on the importance of schedules in the process of reinforcement of the behaviour. A person with autism needs the schedules, and great care is to be taken for the proper planning of the schedules of reinforcement.
5. This theory advocated the avoidance of punishment for unlearning the undesirable behaviour and for shaping the desirable behaviour. Operant conditioning experiments suggested appropriate behaviour to punishment in the form of rewarding appropriate behaviour (*e.g.* differential reinforcement techniques) and ignoring the inappropriate behaviour for its gradual extinction.
6. In its most effective application, theory of operant conditioning has contributed a lot towards the development of programmed instruction and teaching machines, such as
   - Practice should take the form of question (stimulus) – answer (response) frames which expose the student to the subject in gradual steps.
   - Require that the learner make a response for every frame and receive immediate feedback.
   - Try to arrange the difficulty of the questions so

the response is always correct and hence a positive reinforcement.

- Ensure that good performance in the lesson is paired with secondary reinforcers such as verbal praise, prizes and good grades.

Principles

1. Behaviour that is positively reinforced will reoccur; intermittent reinforcement is particularly effective.
2. Information should be presented in small amounts so that responses can be reinforced ('shaping').
3. Reinforcement will generalise across similar stimulus ('stimulus generalisation').

ABA methodologies are grounded in the well-established principles and operant conditioning. In his 'verbal behaviour' book Skinner elaborated on the difference between a traditional or common-sense understanding of language and his behavioural analysis. Skinner's analysis of verbal behaviour as a basis for assessment and intervention programme for children with autism. Overall Skinner's principles originating from operant conditioning have benefitted greatly to children with autism:

II. THE OPERANT CONDITIONING PARADIGM

Operant conditioning refers to increasing or decreasing the probability of a response/behaviour in a particular stimulus environment by presenting a reinforcement by presenting a reinforcement or punishment following the response. The term 'operant' indicates that the organism operates on its environment to generate a consequent behaviour.

The basic process of operant conditioning has been derived from the works of an American Psychologist, Edward L. Thorndike. Later on B.F. Skinner distinguished between respondent conditioning and operant conditioning. The theory of B.F. Skinner is based upon the idea that learning is a function of change in overt behaviour. Changes in behaviour are the result of an individual's response to events (stimuli) that occur in the environment. A response produces a consequence such as defining a word, hitting a ball, or solving a math problem. When a particular stimulus-response (S-R) pattern is reinforced (rewarded), the individual is conditioned to respond. The distinctive characteristic of operant conditioning relative to previous forms of behaviourism (*e.g.* Thorndike, Hall) is that the organism can emit responses instead of only eliciting response due to an external stimulus.

Skinner designed a special apparatus known as Skinner's box. To begin with, Skinner, in one of his experiments, placed a hungry rat in the Skinner box. In this experiment pressing the bar in a desirable way by the rat could result in the production of click sound and presence of a food pallet. The click sound acted as a cue or signal indicating to the rat that if it responds by going to the food cup, it will be rewarded. The rat was rewarded for each of his proper attempts for pressing the lever. The lever press response having been rewarded, was repeated and when it occurred, it was again rewarded which further increased the probability of the repetition of the lever press response and so on. In this way, ultimately, the rat learned the art of pressing the lever as desired by the experimenter.

The important thing in the mechanism of operant conditioning is the emitting of a desired response and its proper management through suitable reinforcement. The subsequent reinforcement gradually conditions the organism to emit the desired response and thus learn the desired act.

Analysing Examples of Operant Conditioning

There are five basic process in operant conditioning:

1. Positive reinforcement,
2. Negative reinforcement,
3. Response cost,
4. Punishment, and
5. Extinction.

Rules in Analysing Examples

The following questions can help in determining whether operant conditioning has occurred:

(*a*) What behaviour in the example was increased or decreased?

(*b*) Was the behaviour increased (if yes, the process has to be either positive or negative reinforcement) or decreased (if the behaviour was decreased the process is either response cost of punishment)?

(*c*) What was the consequence/stimulus that followed the behaviour in the example?

(*d*) Was the consequence/stimulus added or removed? If added the process was either positive reinforcement or punishment. If it was subtracted, the process was either negative reinforcement or response cost.

Our knowledge about operant conditioning has greatly influenced educational practices. In operant conditioning, it is possible to speed up the process of achieving a target behaviour by reinforcing approximations of the target behaviour, through the process of shaping.

III. REINFORCER: POSITIVE AND NEGATIVE

Skinner has emphasised the role of reinforcement in learning. The fundamental principles of operant conditioning is that if organism performs behaviour and receives a reinforcement, then the probability of occurrence of that behaviour in future is increased. Reinforcers maintain the behaviour. Reinforcement is used to strengthen S-R connection and increases the probability of learning a task. It provides a motivation for learning and thus is significant in learning.

A reinforcer is the stimulus whose presentation or removal increases the probability of a response re-occurring. It could be primary reinforcers, *e.g.* food or secondary reinforcers, *e.g.* praise. Reinforcer are basically two in nature:

1. Positive reinforcer, and
2. Negative reinforcer.

Positive Reinforcer

A positive reinforcer is any stimulus the introduction or presentation of which increases the likelihood of a particular behaviour. The word positive has two cues associated with it. First, a positive or pleasant stimulus is used in the process, and second, the reinforcer is added (*i.e.* 'positive' as in + sign for addition).

Negative Reinforcer

A negative reinforcer is any stimulus the removal or withdrawal of which increases the likelihood of a particular behaviour. The word negative has two cues associated with it. First, a negative or aversive stimulus is used in the process and second the reinforcer is subtracted (*i.e.* 'negative' as in – sign for subtraction).

According to the operant conditioning the reinforcement should be pleasant in nature. Positive and negative reinforcements both strengthen or increases reoccurring of the desirable behaviour. Whether behaviour's response is positively or negatively reinforcing depends on the effect it has on behaviour. Positive reinforcement results better for learning, a new response or maintaining a present response; whereas negative reinforcement results better for getting people to avoid some undesirable responses that have been performing frequently. It strengthens not making that responses. Negative reinforcement is not the same as punishments. Negative reinforcements like positive reinforcement increases or strengthens a behaviour punishment on the other hand decreases or weakens behaviour.

IV. GENERALISATION AND TRANSFER

A. Generalisation

Generalisation is the process whereby a skill taught in one situation can be applied in other environments.

Stimulus Generalisation (Similar Stimulus – Same Response)

Occurs when response is triggered by anything resembling the original stimulus.

Response Generalisation (Same Stimulus – Responds in a Number of Different Ways).

Once a response or a number of responses have been learned to a stimulus, a performer will read to the same stimulus by responding in a number of different ways.

B. Transfer

Definition

Transfer of learning is where the learning of one skill/task has an effect on the learning of another skill/task.

Types of Transfer

Proactive Transfer

The performance of one skill is to influence a new skill yet to be learned *e.g.* forward roll – tumble turn.

Retroactive Transfer

The performance of one skill is to influence the performance of a previously learned skill *e.g.* badminton drive – tennis forehand.

Positive Transfer

The knowledge of performance of one skill can help the learning of another skill *e.g.* throwing a ball – badminton clear.

Negative Transfer

The knowledge of one skill can hinder the learning of another skill *e.g.* the use of wrist inplaying a forehand drive in squash compared to a tennis ground strike.

Zero Transfer

Whereby the learning of one skill has no effect on the learning of another skill *e.g.* a lofted pass in football – breast stroke, arm action.

Bilateral Transfer

Whereby transfer occurs between limbs, *e.g.* taking a corner kick with your right foot and then your left foot.

C. Facilitating Generalisation or Transfer of Skills

Generalising a skill (across setting, persons, situation and time) is often a problem for individuals with autism. Although they may be able to acquire a skill in one situation, the performance of a skill in multiple setting does not transfer readily for individuals with autism. After a skill has been acquired in one setting, then the skill needs to be performed in different settings or environments with the instructor present to cue as needed.

For Example:

To teach a child to generalise the principle of walking across the street, it must be taught in many different locations. If he/she is taught in only one location, the child with ASD will think that the rule only applies to one specific place.

I. *Form a Behavioural Perspective*

1. Reinforce the performance of social skills in the natural environment.
2. Train with multiple persons and multiple setting.
3. Ensure the presence and delivery of natural reinforces (positive experiences) for the performance of social skills.
4. Practice the skill in natural environment.
5. Fade prompts as quickly as possible.
6. Provide multiple scenarios and examples for social rules and concepts.
7. Teach self monitoring strategies.
8. Provide 'booster sessions' or extra practice opportunities.

II. *Cognitive Perspective*

1. Encourage application of skills in multiple situations (have the child brain storm other situation).
2. Increase mastery of skill performance.
3. Encourage and facilitate an interest in interacting with others and developing relationships.
4. Build self-efficacy related to social performance.
5. Provide information on why the skill is useful.

V. SPECIFIC TECHNIQUES

There are various methods of intervention:

Applied Behaviour Analysis (ABA)

Applied behaviour analysis (ABA) is the application of behavioural principles to shape behaviours and teach new skills. Applied behaviour analysis is based on the principles of behaviour modification as derived from the work of B.F. Skinner and other behavioural scientists. It was originally developed in the 1960s by Ivar Lovaas, a Norwegian psychologist. The practice of ABA has continued to evolve ever since.

Definitions of ABA vary greatly, as do practices that fall under the heading of ABA. A common definition for ABA is: Applied Behaviour Analysis (ABA) is a systematic process of studying and modifying observable behaviour through a manipulation of the environment. Its principles are derived from extensive basic research.

Range of ABA Practice

The range of practice under the heading of ABA has evolved over the past 30 years and now varies from traditional practices to contemporary practices.

Traditional ABA practice is characterised by highly structured, adult-directed teaching referred to as Discrete Trial Instruction or Training (DTI or DTT) that focusses on teaching correct responses in regimental teaching. Contributions of traditional ABA include the benefit of breaking tasks down into defined steps (task analysis), the importance of using a hierarchy of prompts and prompt fading, and systematically measuring and tracking progress. However, traditional ABA practices are typically not informed by research on child and human development; use primarily adult-child (1:1) teaching formats to the exclusion of social instruction in various settings; do not take into account a child's developmental profile; and teach skills that do not necessarily focus on the core social-communicative and relationship challenges faced by children with ASD.

Contemporary ABA practice is characterised by more flexible, naturalistic teaching (incidental teaching) in natural routines and activities that focus on social initiation and spontaneity in daily routines and activities. Based on the significant limitations of traditional ABA practice, many ABA practitioners have moved away from highly structured, prescriptive practice to practices that have a much greater focus on social communication across a variety of social settings, and the need to determine functions of behaviour to replace less desirable behaviour. In many ways, contemporary ABA practice, such as Discrete Trial Instruction (DTI), incidental teaching, Pivotal Response Training (PRT), positive behavioural support, Early Intensive Behavioural Intervention (EIBI) and Verbal Behaviour Intervention (VBI) is more similar to developmentally based approaches (*e.g.* SCERTS, RDI and Floor-time) than it is to traditional ABA practice. The development of contemporary ABA practice has been heavily influenced by research on language and play development in typical children, with an emphasis on individualised and positive approaches to understand and address problem behaviour.

Skill Focussed in ABA Programmes

ABA programme focus on the development of comprehensive skills including language skills, social skills, play or leisure skills, motor skills, academic skills and self-help skills. Language skills are critical for independent functioning, cognitive growth and social development. Social, play and leisure skills are also important and enhance a child's quality of life. Self-help skills build independence and academic skills help a child access the general education curriculum.

Basic Principles of ABA

A sound ABA programme should include four components: (1) Discrete Trial Instruction (DTI), (2) chaining procedures, (3) natural environmental training and (4) incidental teaching.

ABA programmes emphasise the importance of looking at the ABC's (antecedents, behaviours and consequences) of behaviours, teaching new behaviours and developing systematic instructional plans to teach new skills. ABA is the best method for managing undesirable and aberrant behaviours such as: self-injurious, repetitive, ritualistic, aggressive and disruptive behaviours; and promotes alternative pro-social behaviours simultaneously.

Skills that are to be promoted are broken down into small sequential steps. The ABC principles of behaviour intervention are used to teach the child each step:

A (antecedent)	– Each instruction is given clearly, in as few words as possible. Assistance is provided; for example prompting through demonstration or physically guiding.
B (behaviour)	– An appropriate behaviour is observed.
C (consequence)	– A consequence is an outcome that will reward the child and increase the likelihood that the behaviour will be repeated again in the future, also called a positive reinforcer.

This 'ABC' process is repeated frequently for each behaviour both in structured teaching situations and in the course of everyday activities.

1. Instructions are given to emphasise metacognition (learning how to learn). In this case learning how to listen, to watch, to initiate, to ask and do.
2. As the child's learned behaviours improve, the structured guidance is systematically reduced and the prompts are used less frequently and eventually faded out. Thus so that the child learns to perform the trained behaviour independently.
3. It is also important to change the context of teaching (different people giving the antecedent, more people around, different situations, etc.) in order to generalise the learned behaviours.
4. When each behaviour consisting of single sequential steps are acquired, the person is taught to combine them to produce more complex behaviours.
5. Problematic behaviours are not reinforced, instead the child is consistently redirected to engage in appropriate behaviour.
6. The child's response during each step is meticulously recorded. The information is later used to determine if the child is progressing at an acceptable rate. If progress is not satisfactory, the learning steps are analysed for possible flaws and the programme modified.

Principles of ABA are being widely used all over the world.

Verbal Behaviour Analysis (VBA)

Verbal behaviour analysis, a speciality within the field of Applied Behaviour Analysis (ABA). B.F. Skinner extended operant conditioning to verbal behaviour in his book *Verbal Behaviour* (1957) thus providing a functional analysis of language meaning that use of a word can functionally represent more than one thing. These were termed verbal operants (*e.g.* mand (request), tact (labels), echoic, receptive identification, intraverbal etc.). Thus the word 'apple' can represent a request or mand given a state of deprivation or label when stated in the presence of the item. This led to the application of the analysis of verbal behaviour into an ABA programme has become more popular in recent years and is based on research. It is important to conceptualise that the use of verbal behaviour analysis is not distinctively different from ABA but rather a component of ABA programming.

'Language' – Form of Verbal Behaviour

In his book 'verbal behaviour' Skinner proposes that language is a form of behaviour and like other behaviours caused by environmental variables such as reinforcement, motivation, extinction and punishment. The commonly held view of language assumes that it is caused by biological and cognitive variables.

Amongst children with pervasive developmental disorders, some children appear to have normal language development and then lose it. Others do not develop language at all. Still others have delayed language development. The children who have a delay or deviance in language acquisition oftendevelop inappropriate or negative behaviour. Behaviour analysts believe that the connection to language is often missed or overlooked. For instance a child who wants to play with a toy may push another child in order to get the toy. The pushing behaviour may be treated through extinction or some other punishment procedure. However, that will not provide the child with the means of getting the toy, which was the real reason behind the 'violent behaviour' of pushing other children. So the punishment may not work long-term or some other inappropriate behaviour may take its place.

Most non-verbal children develop forms of communication that has been shaped over the years. Self-injurious behaviour, screaming, hitting and other inappropriate behaviours may serve as verbal behaviour for such children. It is necessary to study and understand the antecedents and consequences of such behaviours in order to develop appropriate language intervention programmes.

Behavioural Classification of Language in VBA

In the practice of verbal behaviour, language is analysed by its formal and functional properties. The formal properties are grammar and systanx (sentence structure), and also include articulation, intonation, pitch and so on. The functional properties consists of the situation under which responses occur. Skinner's analysis of verbal behaviour led to a classification of language that permits the identification of these different functional types. Very briefly these are the following:

Mand	Asking for reinforcers that you want. A tendency to ask for a dog because you want one.
Tact	Naming or identifying objects, actions, events, etc. A tendency to say 'dog' because you see a dog.
Receptive	Following or complying with the instructions of others. A tendency to touch a-picture of a dog when asked to touch the dog.
Echoic	Repeating what is heard. A tendency to say 'dog' after someone else says 'dog'.
Imitation	Copying someone's motor movements. A tendency to clap after someone else claps.
RFFC	Identifying specific items when given some description (function, features or class) of the item. A tendency to touch a dog when someone says 'Which one barks?'
Intraverbal	Answering questions or conversations where your words are controlled by other's words. A tendency to say 'dog' when someone else says 'Lassie'.
Textual	Reading written words. A tendency to say 'dog' because you see the written word 'dog.'
Writing	Writing and spelling words when spoken to you. A tendency to write 'dog' because you hear it spoken.

Verbal behaviour analysis uses errorless teaching, keeping learner errors low and success and motivation high. VBA also encourages generalisation by keeping tasks mixed and varied. VBA promotes the use of sign language rather than the use of PECs. Finally, VBA places great store by Natural Environment Training (NET) *i.e.* is teaching in the natural environment.

Discrete Trial Training (DTT)

The discrete trial is the primary teaching method for a number of the behaviourally-based interventions used in teaching children with autism. In fact, Discrete Trial Training (DTT) is often synonymous with applied behavioural analysis (ABA), though that is a practice that should probably be discouraged, as they are two very different beasts.

Children with autism often face many deficits and difficulties in learning. Discrete trial training can help to compensate for these difficulties.

- DTT tasks are broken down into short, simple trials and increases child's attention.
- DTT attempts to build motivation by rewarding performance of desired behaviours.
- In DTT the presented stimuli are clear and relatively consistent.
- DTT programmes are designed to change over time, in content and context to strengthen generalisation.
- DTT teaches skills and behaviours explicitly to enhance cause-effect learning
- The instructions given in DTT are simple, concrete and clearly provide only the most salient information to overcome communication deficiency.
- DTT designed to avoid problems in perspective taking and understanding of social and behavioural expectations.

1. ***Parts of Discrete Trial Training***

A discrete trial is a single cycle of a behaviourally-based instruction routine. A particular trial may be repeated several times in succession, several times a day, over several days until the skill is mastered. There are four parts and an optimal fifth, to a discrete trial.

- The *Discriminative Stimulus* (S^D): The instruction or environmental cue to which the teacher would like to child to respond.
- The *Prompting Stimulus* (S^P): A prompt or cue from the teacher to help the child respond correctly (optional).
- The *Response* (R): The skill or behaviour that is the target of the instruction, or a portion thereof
- The *Reinforcing Stimulus* (S^R): A reward designed to motivate the child to respond and respond correctly.
- The *Inter-trial Interval* (ITI): A brief-pause between consecutive trials. The parts of the discrete trial are often represented symbolically like so:

$$S^D \rightarrow R \rightarrow S^R \rightarrow ITI$$
$$(S^P)$$

Essentially this illustrates the order of a discrete trial. First comes the teacher's instruction (S^D). If the teacher thinks the child may need some help responding correctly, she will give him a little prompt, cue, as model to help him and (S^P). Then, either with help or without, the child gives some response to the instruction (R). If he responds correctly, or close to correctly, the teacher might give him some reward or praise to encourage him (S^R). If the child responds incorrectly she might correct him, and then give him another chance, at the most, two incorrect responses. After that is completed, a pause between each trial-long enough so each trial is distinct but not so long that the child loses focus or begins alternative behaviours. The intertrial interval can last between one and three seconds.

2. *The Acquisition Process*

Within each programme there will be a specific target. This is referred to as the 'item on acquisition' and there is only one item on acquisition within any one programme at any one time. Each programme has a 'current items lists'. This contains a numbered list of all the items that are going to be targetted within that programme. Items are targetted using a systematic approach based on collected data.

MT – (DT) – (ET) – RR

- MT → Mass trial (targetted item on its own)
- DT → Distractor trial (neutral distractor)
- ET → Expanded trial (intermixing with mastered items)
- RR → Random rotation (other mastered items)

During the acquisition process, the activity starts a series of three to five successive discrete trials in MT and DT. Then a series of six to eight successive discrete trial in Expanded Trial (ET) and five to seven successive trials in random rotation (RR). The ET and RR are optional and depends on the programme and the child's rate of learning.

3. *Mastery Criteria*

Mastery criteria relates to the results of the data gathered at each sitting. The mastery criteria refers to the series of results of a child must score in order to move on to the next change in the acquisition process or for the introduction of a new item.

A typical mastery criteria would be:

X 3 successive 100% @ MT across 2 therapists, across 2 days
X 3 successive 100% @ DT across 2 therapists, across 2 days
X 3 successive 100% @ RR across 2 therapists, across 2 days

An item considered 'mastered' once it has reached the mastery criteria for that particular programme.

4. *Teaching Complex Behaviours*

While most of the discussion so far has centred around simple behaviours – eliciting a choice, a particular phrase etc., many of the behaviours that a child needs to be taught are more complex made up of many such simpler skills.

There are a pair of techniques, shaping and chaining, can be used to teach more complex behaviours. Shaping begins with a step analysis, chaining links the component of behaviours by forward or backward chaining.

Lovaas Method

The Lovaas method is an early intensive behaviour therapy approach for children with autism and other related disorder. It is also known as the UCLA (University of California, Los Angles) programme by Dr. Ivan Lovaas, home-based behavioural intervention and UCLA model of applied behaviour analysis as developed in the Lovaas Institute of Early Intervention. It is based on extensive clinical experience and research carried out over more than 30 years.

In the late 60s and 70s Lovaas worked with institutionalised, non-verbal children who had been diagnosed as autistic. He concentrated on verbal communication using the strategies of applied behaviour analysis. At the time Lovaas work was criticised by colleagues advocating the psychodynamic approach, because most of the children lost their verbal skills when the programme ceased and they returned to institutional life. However, those who moved back with parents, who wanted to be informed about the treatment, did much better. This led to an increased importance of the role of parents in the education process.

Home-Based Programme

Lovaas and his colleagues recommended that treatment should begin as early as possible, preferably before the child is five years old and, ideally, before the child reaches three and a half years.

The home-based programme consists of 40 hours a week of intensive therapy. The therapy is on one-to-one basis for six to eight hours per day, five to seven days a week, for two or more years. Teaching session usually last two to three hours with breaks. The programme team which normally consists of at least three persons and have all undergone a full training programme.

Family participation is a very important element of the treatment. All skills are broken down into small tasks that are achievable and taught in a very structured manner and accompanied by lots of praise and reinforcement. Aggressive or self-stimulatory behaviours are reduced or replaced by ignoring them or by introducing more socially acceptable forms of behaviour. In the 60s and 70s aversive procedures had been used by behaviour analysts. In his early work Lovaas defended its use in situations when a child used self-injurious or self-stimulatory behaviours. He contended that aversive procedures constituted no more than 1% of the typical interactions in his programme and that they are not generally required after the first few weeks. The UCLA project no longer employs aversive procedures.

The intervention programme progresses very gradually from teaching basic self-help and language skills to teaching non-verbal and verbal imitation skills, and establishing the beginning of toy play. Second stage teaches expressive and early abstract language and interactive play with peers. In more advanced stages of the intervention the child can be taught at home and school.

Benefits of Lovaas Method

Lovaas closely supervised the one-to-one home-based programme. The results were published in 1987 and caused interest as up until then there had been no studies to show that behavioural strategies could present such positive results.

Lovaas compared three groups of 20 children:

1. The experimental group of children who received 40 hours a week of treatment.
2. A first control group who received 10 hours behavioural treatment together with a variety of treatments from other sources such as those provided by small special educational classes.
3. A second control group who received no behavioural treatment.

Lovaas described his findings from the experimental group as follows:

(*a*) A recoverable group of individuals, who, following intervention, no longer demonstrated the characteristic of autism (47% of children),

(*b*) An intermediate group (40%) who made substantial progress but who still displayed autistic characteristics, and

(*c*) A small number (10%) who received little or no benefit from the intervention.

The results also showed that those children who followed the programme for two years or more gained on average 30 IQ points compared with the other two group who made no IQ gains.

A following study carried out in 1993 indicated that the majority had maintained their gains into adolescence. There have been numerous articles and critiques written on this topic over the last 20 years and many arguments as to the validity of Lovaas findings.

Summary

Many of the behavioural approaches for autism are derived from the works of parlor, Watson and Skinner, the founders of behaviourist psychology. Skinner found that the human response as voluntarily controlled. Skinner determined that a desired behaviours can be achieved by rewarding a random behaviour that leads to desired behaviour. This process is called "operant conditioning". Ivar Lovaas applied these theories to children with autism in a form what is called applied behaviour analysis. His work provided a foundation for other professionals to develop various ABA therapies and other teaching methods for children with autism. Among many methods available for treatment and education of people with autism. ABA has become medley accepted as an effective treatment. B.F. Skinner extended operant conditioning to verbal behaviour in his book Verbal Behaviour (1957), and Verbal Behaviour Analysis (VBA) emerged from Skinners proposes that language is a form of behaviour.

4

Communication Centred Therapy

I. THE ENHANCEMENT OF COMMUNICATION TO DEAL WITH THE VERBAL, NON-VERBAL AND BEHAVIOUR DIFFICULTIES OF CHILDREN WITH ASD

Generally babies came into the world eager to communicate. They are 'pre-programmed', ready to soak up what they see and hear and make sense of it. Children with autism may not be as eager to communicate. They may not be ready to learn the things which other babies learn naturally and therefore do not have the chance to 'tune in' to language in the same way. They find it very hard to make sense of the things which happen around them. Words may mean very little to them and they may be unable to link what they see with things being said to them. Young children with autism not only have difficulty making sense of words but also in 'reading' non-verbal messages in facial expressions and gestures. Communication problems are central to autism.

Most learners with autism who can hear have a good – perhaps excellent – ability to receive or take in and store verbal information. However auditory processing discrepancies can result in many learning and behaviour problems. They need access to verbal information in a form they can understand. Adaptations and many positive language experiences will most likely result in better understanding and meaningful use. Therefore special care must be taken to know what each person understands and how to provide the messages.

They need extra time to process the auditory information and produce a response. Stop talking and wait expectantly for at least

30 seconds before repeating or rephrasing the question or direction.

A. General Recommendations

Many of the children with autism understand a lot of what they hear when they are listening or attending. However, they do have a variety of problems *i.e.* they are frequently 'tuned out' and therefore miss out on some of the information or gaps in their knowledge of word meanings and concepts or they understand language in literal or concrete terms or words that depend on the context for meaning.

The following general techniques are helpful:

1. *Multi-model Communication*: Illustrate key words, sequences, and outcomes while speaking. Visual information is more concrete and enduring. Draw pictures, write words, or point out the learner's visual communication system. Make critical information visual.
2. *Minimise Direct Questions*: It is important to minimise use of direct questions. Ask questions only when there are real choices and when the answer is not known.
   e.g.
   Ineffective: "Are you ready to work"?
   [Learner's perspective: Oh, god! I have a choice. I don't really like doing that work, and I still want to watch the leaves bloming in the tree. I'll just stay here.]
   Effective: "It will be time to work when the bell rings".
   [Learner's perspective: Okay, a few more minutes to watch the leaves, then back to work.]
3. *Speak Positively*: Tell the learner what to do?
   e.g.
   Ineffective: "Don't get out of the chair".
   [Learner's perspective: Oh! I have to stay in this chair always or did he say get out of the chair? Okay, I'll stand up.]
   Learner's often do exactly what they were told not to do. It could be that some do not process the first part of the sentence and hear only the end.

Effective: Say, 'sit in the chair'; or "sit in the chair until we finish colouring".

4. *Speak Literally and Very Specifically*:

   e.g.

   Ineffective: 'Give me the cow' – when directing a learner to identify pictures.

   [Learner's perspective: I don't see a cow, couldn't lift it if it were here. Guess, I'll just sit here until she tells me to do something I can do.]

   Effective: 'Give me the picture of cow'.

5. *Use Exaggerated Facial Expressions and Abundant Gestures*: Using abundant, exaggerated facial expression and bodily gesture is crucial in fostering language acquisition. Movement and gestures in both the instructor and the child will encourage speech. Capture the child's attention and support the meaning of the words using.

6. *Use Language that is Simple, Clear and Concise.* Verbalise basic information simply, briefly and clearly. Children with autism can only comprehend a limited amount of language directed at them. It is best to be concise loading too many directions and explanations create frustrations and confusion. Express a complete thought to clarify the message. Avoid verbal – overloaded.

   e.g.

   Ineffective: 'Find coat.'

   [Learner's perspective: Which coat? Find. Is it lost? Okay! The coat is over there. I found it. Let me wait I don't know what to do.]

   Effective: "Put on your red coat. Then we can walk to the park."

7. *Speak at a Normal Rate*: Speak in full sentences and at a normal rate of speed so the child will be able to understand. When introducing a new concept or a critical piece of information:

   - Pause briefly to separate the relevant words from ongoing conversations.
   - Speak a bit more slowly than usual.
   - Pair key words with visual references (words or line drawings).

8. *Teach the Meaning of Rules and Directions*: Be prepared to teach and highlight the meaning of directions, both

verbally and visually. Then provide assistance to carry out the directions quickly to ensure that the correct response is firmly associated with the directions.

e.g.

A tape line on the floor between the door way to define a rule, "stay in the living room".

9. *Be as Neutral as Possible When Giving Directions*: The tone of voice, a facial expression, or the difference of a word can change the meaning of a question, direction or statement when giving a direction, state what needs to be done and avoid challenges. Individuals tend to become defensive or upset and try to avoid or do the opposite of what is asked when directions are given in a threatening manner.
10. *Model the Expression of Feelings*: Individuals with autism have great difficulty is recognising feelings of others and expressing their own feelings. Model the expression of feelings as emotional situations are explained. Do not discount or ignore feelings even when the learner's expressions do not match with the situations. Rather, provide a more typical model.

    e.g.

    If the learner laughs hysterically when a friend is hurt, look sad and say, "Mary feel and hurt her knee. She feels bad. I feel sorry because her knee hurts."
11. *Give Adequate Information*: Tell learners in advance what is going to happen next. If there are changes, inform them and involve them in plans. Let the learners know what will happen and what behaviour is expected. Use language, pictures, and gestures they understand. Daily schedule boards and sequence routines made with charts, check-off sheets and pictures are concrete ways to provide information.
12. *Avoid Threats and Reprimands*: Threats provide negative responses. They are a negative way to give consequences *e.g.* say, "be quiet, then we will go to the playground". Avoid saying, "if you are not quiet, you won't get to go to the park".

    Also, reprimands have little meaning to most children with autism and will not change the behaviour. For *e.g.* avoid saying, "I've told you not to go into the street a hundred times." Say, "The rule is, ride on the bike sidewalks."

Learners with autism need clear and understandable information in order to participate successfully in the community. They need access to the language.

B. Communication to Deal Behaviour Difficulties

Reflective listening is used when a person has a problem and anxiety is accelerating to moderately high level. This strategy.

- Recognises that a problem exists.
- Expresses concern and establishes a mutually respectful relationship.
- Identifies and clarifies the problem.
- Provides labels (the language) for the problem, the feelings, and the solutions.
- Defuses frustration and anxiety.
- Sets the stage for solving problems.

This strategy involves the following five steps:

1. Recognise and identify the subtle, non-verbal cues (behavioural signals) that indicate the presence of a problem, a need, emotion, or feelings that need to be communicated.
2. Quickly scan the environment for cues to interpret the cause of the problem.
3. Tentatively verbalise the feeling and the problem. ("You look hot and thirsty. Do you need a drink?")
   - A hesitant statement is respectful and appropriate because an interpreter can never be totally, certain of another person's feelings or needs.
   - Be as precise and descriptive as possible when labelling feelings and emotions.
4. Pause for acknowledgement. Acknowledgement may be made in a variety of ways: for *e.g.* the learner may make feeling eye contact or become very still and the signs of stress may begin to decrease. If the statement did not accurately express the feeling or need, the stress will

continue to escalate. In that case, make another effort to clarify the situation.

5. Suggest a way for the problem to be resolved, and provide assistance to solve it quickly. Because most problems can be solved by asking for help or for clarification, it is appropriate to provide a cue for how to communicate the message.

This reflective listening strategy can be modified to match specific situations. For *e.g.* reduce the number of words for a younger or less sophisticated learner, and use fewer words if the stress level increases.

II. HEARING AND LISTENING IN CHILDREN WITH ASD

To become a good learner, one has to become a good listener. Hearing and listening are not one and the same. There is a huge difference between the two. Listening is a specialised form of hearing. Listening, not hearing, is the primary function of the ear.

Distinction between Hearing and Listening

- Hearing is a passive process. It is merely detecting the sound around us.
- Listening is an active process. It requires the conscious desire to determine the meaning of what we hear.

A. Auditory Problems in Autism

Children with autism rarely have hearing problems but tend to display abnormal listening patterns. Many people with autism often has Central Auditory Processing Disorder (CAPD). Auditory problems in autism include inability to filter auditory information, hypersensitivity, hyposensitivity, inability to modulate certain sounds, delays in auditory processing and others. These problems may be covered by a single definition – auditory dysfunction. This dysfunction is often undetected as a conventional hearing test may not show any problems, especially in older children and adults who have acquired strategies to cope with their difficulties, such as blocking out sounds.

Recently a subtype of auditory dysfunction has been signed out and described as Central Auditory Processing Disorder (CAPD). CAPD as defined as a neurological dysfunction responsible for impairments of neural pathways of the brain that link the ear with the central auditory system when the ear works properly but the parts of the brain that interpret and analyse the auditory information do not.

Some indicators of CAPD are:

- May seem deaf at some occasions but hears the slightest sounds at other occasions.
- Covers bars even if there are no loud sounds.
- Produces sounds (banging door, tapping things, making vocalisations, etc.).
- Cannot concentrate in noisy environments.
- Speech problems.
- A very light sleeper.

People with autism often suffer unbearable pain because of they have multiple sensitivities. These problems can leave the person unable to concentrate properly as extraneous sounds constantly impinge upon them. Thus when listening to others the person with autism may hear a single word or two or even a simple sentence but longer sentences may be 'broken up' by intruding background noises and the meaning lost.

Normally, when people listen predominantly with their ears, the sounds are filtered to reduce its intensity. Also, they are able to filter out all the background noises, so that they can tune into what is really important. Many autistic people do not have the ability to filter out background noises and tune into what really matters.

B. The Tomatis Method

French Otolaryngologist and Psychologist Alfred Tomatis conducted research in the field of auditory processing problems that resulted in his theory – "The Tomatis effect". Tomatis's 'listening therapy' greatly improved the life of many autistic people, by attenuating the symptoms. It is often in conjunction with other therapies. The Tomatis programme tries to help autistic children to develop self-listening to foster communication. The programme consists of two stages:

1. Auditory *i.e.* receptive, when the person is trained to develop better listening skills.
2. Audio-vocal *i.e.* expressive, when the person is trained to develop voice of good quality and tone to maintain listening skills.

C. Berard Method

Guy Berard, a French Otolaryngologist, originally trained by Tomatis, disagreed with his teacher in a number of points and developed his own approach to the problem. In contrast to Tomatis, who assumed psychological causes of the disorder, Berard suggested biological causes. Berard developed Auditory Integration Training (AIT) and special device Audiokinetron. AIT is based on two assumptions:

1. Behaviour is a direct result of how well a person hears.
2. The hearing mechanism can be retrained. As a result, improved hearing leads to improved behaviour.

D. The Listening Programme (TLP)

An alternative to the Tomatis method is the listening programme (TLP) which is home-based sound stimulation programme. TLP is based on the same scientific rationale as Tomatis and uses similar filtration techniques which are programmed on the CDs. Sometimes TLP is used in combination with Neuro Developmental Therapy (NDT) so that the body is stimulated through both sound and sensory input. The neuro development therapy involves a programme of movements designed to retrace motor development as it ideally should have been experienced and has been shown to be of considerable benefit to children with autism.

III. COMMUNICATION DEVELOPMENT AND CHARACTERISTICS IN ASD INCLUDING SEMANTIC-PRAGMATIC DEFICIT AND HYPERLEXIA

Communication is an active, intentional and two way process. The speaker intentionally transmits information (message) and the listener intentionally receives it and subsequently they may exchange their roles. It is also possible to communicate without intending to do so *e.g.* displeasure, which we want to hide, gets expressed through eyes, body postures, tone, etc. In order for us to effectively communicate we need skills in multiple areas, including verbal and non-verbal areas.

People with autism are characterised by deficits in the ability to communicate. They experience difficulties in understanding and developing functional and meaningful communication. People with autism may not have sufficient underestimating of their own experience and feelings, of those of other people, and of the relationship between themselves and others, to fully grasp the significance and need of communication.

A. Communication Development and Characteristics in ASD

The most intensive period of speech and lanaguage development is during first three years of life, a period when the brain is developing and maturing. These skills appears to develop best in a world that is rich with sounds, sights and consistent exposure to the speech and language of others. At the root of this development is the desire to communicate or interact with the world. The quality of social communicative interaction is remarkedly different in autism.

Children with an ASD often fail to communicate using speech or any other type of language, for *e.g.* eye contact, hand gestures, body language. If a child does not wish to communicate intentionally (a trait of ASD) they will not explore their ability to vocalise, learn new sounds or listen to the language spoken around them.

A child with an ASD may not see any reason to communicate with other people, also remove themselves from situations that require communication. The communication problems of autism vary, depending upon the intellectual and social development of the individual. Some may be unable to speak, whereas others may have rich vocabularies and are able to talk about topics of interest in great depth. Despite this variation, the majority of autistic individuals have little or no problem with pronunciation. Those who can speak often say things that have no content or information. Others use echolalia, a repetition of something previously heard, it could be immediate echolalia or delayed echolalia. Some children may use stock phrases such as, 'My name is Tom' to start a conversation, even when speaking with friends or family. Still others may repeat learned scripts such as those heard during television commercials. Some individuals with higher intelligence may be able to speak in depth about topics they are interested but are unable to engage in an interactive conversation on those topics.

Most autistic individuals do not make eye contact and have poor attention duration. They are often unable to use gestures either as a primary means of communication, as in sign language, or to assist verbal communication, such as pointing to an object they want. Some children speak in a high-pitched voice or use robot-like speech. They are often unresponsive to the speech of others and may not respond to their own names. As a result, some are mistakenly thought to have a hearing problem. The correct use of pronouns is also a problem for autistic individuals.

For many, speech and language develop, to some degree, but not to a normal ability level. This development is usually uneven. Many have good memories for information just heard or seen. Some may be able to read words well before the age five but may not be able to demonstrate understanding of what is read.

Although the cause of speech and language problems in ASD is unknown, many experts believe that the difficulties are caused by a variety of conditions that occur either before, during, or after birth affect brain development. This interferes with an individual's ability to interpret and interact with the world. Some scientists tie the communication problem to a 'theory of mind' or impaired ability to think about thoughts or imagine another individual's state of mind. Along with this is an impaired ability to symbolise both when trying to communicate and in play.

B. Semantic and Pragmatic Difficulties

I. *Semantics*

Semantic is the aspect of language function that relates to understanding the meaning of words, phrases and sentences, and using words appropriately when we speak. Children with semantic difficulties have a very hard time understanding the meaning of words and sentences.

People with semantic processing difficulties have particular trouble with abstract words. They have difficulty with idioms, sayings and slang expressions, often taking them literally or interpreting them oddly. For *e.g.*: when asked if he enjoyed spending time with his friends, a 14 year old child with Aspergers and semantic processing problems replied, "I don't see how you can spend time, and I certainly don't see how you could enjoy it because spending time is not something you can do. You can only actually spend money."

Another difficulty children with semantic problem experience is that they may not be able to identify the key point or topic in a sentence and because of this may suddenly change the subject, very obscurely, apparently thinking they are on the same subject. Here is another real example from a girl aged eleven. Question, "Could you get the book of the shelf and give it to me?" Reply. "The Gulf stream warms the coast line".

Note: Close questioning revealed that the obscure connection here was the continental 'shelf' and the Gulf 'stream'. Her response was related to her deep interest in marine biology and ocean currents.

II. *Pragmatics*

Pragmatics is the area of language function that embraces the use of language in social contexts (knowing what to say, how to say it and when to say it, and how to 'be' with other people).

Children with pragmatic difficulties have great trouble using language socially in ways that are appropriate or typical of children of their age. They often do not understand that we take turns to talk, and they will, 'talk over the top of you' at times, or at other times respond to what you say with inappropriate silences, or in a voice that is too quiet. They may interrupt excessively and talk irrelevantly or about things the listener shows no interest in. Their communicative behaviour often appears rude and inconsiderate.

They often do not assume prior knowledge. For *e.g.*: one boy explained to his car driver in minute detail how to wash a car, wrongly assuming that he needed (and wanted) the information and that he had never washed a car.

On the other hand, they may assume prior knowledge that the listener could not possibly have, and launch into a long disquisition without describing in sufficient detail the participants, location and general background of their story. They can go on far too long telling stories, and include so much detail that the listener becomes disinterested.

Pragmatic skills include:

1. Knowing that you have to answer when a question has been asked;
2. Being able to participate in a conversation by taking it in turns with the other speaker;
3. The ability to notice and respond to the non-verbal aspect of language (reacting appropriately to the other person's body language and 'mood', as well as their words);
4. Awareness that you have to introduce a topic of conversation in order for the listener to fully understand;
5. Knowing which words or what sort of sentence type to use when initiating a consideration or responding to something some one has said;
6. The ability to maintain a topic (or change topic appropriately, or 'interrupt' politely);
7. The ability to maintain appropriate eye-contact (not too much staring, and not too much looking away) during a conversation; and
8. The ability to distinguish how to talk and behave towards different communicative partners (formal with some, informal with others).

III. *Semantic-Pragmatic Language Disorder in Autistic Continuum*

Semantic-Pragmatic Disorder (SPD) was originally defined in the literature on language disorder in 1983, by Rapin and Allen, although at that time it was classified as a syndrome. They referred to a group of children who presented with mild autistic features and specific semantic pragmatic language problems. Some authorities see Semantic-Pragmatic Language Disorder (SPLD) [called Semantic-Pragmatic Disorder (SPD) in some literature) as part of the autism spectrum disorders while others see it purely as a language disorder.

All the children on the autistic continuum including those with core autism have semantic-pragmatic difficulties with language and they should all be viewed in the context of autism. That is they share the same triad of difficulties with sociability, pretence and language.

There is an argument, at least in the early years, particularly for more able children, to use less specific diagnostic labels like autism and simply to describe children who may well-improved dramatically in the pre-school years as falling within the 'autistic continuum' or as having an autism spectrum disorder.

Children with Asperger Syndrome are generally earlier fluent speakers. There seems to be a pay off between early comprehension skills and sociability. As children mature, it is often difficult to specify what label best fits. There is clearly an enormous difference between a child with severe learning difficulties and autism and a child of superior intelligence with a semantic-pragmatic language disorder. When we are describing children on the autistic continuum, we must also be clear in our minds about whether we are simply describing levels of sociability or whether we are also describing more generalised learning difficulty. Two do not necessarily go hand in hand.

It is always necessary to determine whether the child has:

1. Isolated semantic processing difficulties in the autistic spectrum, or
2. Isolated pragmatic processing difficulties in the autistic spectrum, or
3. Combination of semantic pragmatic difficulties in the autistic spectrum, or
4. SPLD in combination with another communication disorder that is not in the autism spectrum, for *e.g.* Apraxia, or
5. SPLD in combination with another that is NOT in the autism spectrum, *e.g.*: Attention Deficit Hyperactivity Disorder (ADHD), or
6. Semantic-pragmatic language disorder.

There are many children with semantic and pragmatic difficulties who don't quite 'fit' into a definite diagnostic category.

C. Hyperlexia

Hyperlexia refers the ability to spell, read, and pronounce words is markedly advance for their age. Usually these kids have easily mastered letters and numbers by the age of two, and by three can read many words. They seem to have a far greater capacity for reading than for spontaneous speech. They may eventually even read and pronounce words at a college level, yet have a difficult time in comprehending the meaning of the words, or how to use them in the right context. These kids are master decoders, but poor interpreters. For *e.g.*: they might read a Harry Potter book with ease, but have great difficulty answering 'why' questions about the book. They love books, words, and may find word play entertaining. However, they find spoken language hard to understand.

Definition

Hyperlexia is a syndrome characterised by an intense fascination with letters or numbers and an advanced reading ability. Hyperlexic children read at levels far beyond those of their age mates and often begin reading at very young ages, sometimes at age two.

Hyperlexic children have excellent visual and auditory memories, which means they easily remember what they see and hear. They use their memory to help them learn language. They will often exhibit echolalia, which is the repetition of phrases and sentences without understanding the meaning. Given their difficulty with spoken language, hyperlexic children rarely initiate conversations.

A. *Hyperlexia in ASD*

The hyperlexic children are known as 'precocious readdress' and are often treated as 'autistic savants'. Many children with autism show the same patterns of hyperlexic, that is, with an ability to decode, but a seeming inability to comprehend. Not all children with autism are hyperlexic but developmental disturbances, especially in the area of language and socialisation, are always present in hyperlexic. The patterns of reading skills that are intact and impaired within the autism population. This is important for number of reasons, including clarifying the definition of hyperlexia, increasing awareness of strengths and weakness of students with autism when it comes to decoding text, from the simple words to the entire concept of reading comprehension, and global comprehension in general.

B. *Characteristics of Hyperlexia and Autism*

Hyperlexia is considered to be part of the autism spectrum disorders and like children with autism, children with hyperlexia have problems in socialising and behaving appropriately. They also exhibit other characteristics of autism:

- Self-Stimulating behaviour
- Ritualistic behaviour
- Concrete and literal thinking
- Difficulty with abstract concepts
- Normal development until 18-24 months followed by regression
- Need to keep routines
- Difficulty transitioning from one activity to another

Additional characteristics of autism includes the following:

- Sensitivity to sounds, smells and touch
- Unusual fears
- Selective listening (may appear to be deaf)

Obviously not all children with ASD have the striking ability to recognise and decode words. Hyperlexia has characteristics similar to autism, behaviour disorder, language disorder, emotional disorder. Attention deficit disorder, hearing impairment, giftedness or paradoxically, mental retardation. To develop effective teaching strategies and more typical childhood development, it is important to differentiate hyperlexia from other disorder. The term 'autism' is being spread too thin, covering all kinds of different disorders which should have their own name.

IV. COMMUNICATION CENTRED TECHNIQUES

Communication and interaction is just as important for children with autism as it is for other children. As the understanding of autism as it is for other children. As the understanding of autism spectrum disorder has grown in recent years, we are better able to use very effective strategies in making communication enjoyable and result oriented. The fruit of past research in autism includes varied interventions, and techniques in the communication domain. For *e.g.*: visually mediated communication; TEACCH; PECS; AIT; ACC etc.

In this section, we briefly explore these techniques:

A. Visually Meditated Communication

Visually meditated communication was developed by Dr. Hogdon, a speech pathologist by profession. Hodgon's initial and primary intervention concern is comprehension. Visual supports are an integral part of the communication circle, enhancing effective receiving, processing, action and expression. Her book "visual strategies for improving communication (1996)" is a must read manual. This book is chock full of examples and illustration, providing clear guidance and direction to all who wish to employ effective strategy to improve communication skills.

Visual Tools

Visual tools are developed as a means to support communication. There are mainly four sections which describes the visual options with pictures and samples as examples. They are:

1. Tools to give information.
2. Aids to give effective directions.
3. Visual strategies to organise the environment.
4. Mediating communication between environments.

These strategies have application for students ranging in ability from severe mental impairment to gifted. Most students will benefit from the concrete structure provided by many of these tools.

1. *Tools to Give Information*: A major function of communication is to give information. Visual aids such as schedules, calendars, mini-schedules, choice boards, and menu, people locators are visual tools whose primary

function is to give information in a concrete visual forms which helps as following:

- Clarifying verbal information
- Provides a concrete way to teach concepts such as time, sequence, cause/effect.
- Gives structure to understand and accept change.
- Supports transitions between activities as locations.
- Gives information in a form that the student can quickly and easily interpret.
- Helps established and maintain attention.

2. *Aids to Give Effective Directions*: One classroom management tools support both routine and unique communications we use during daily activities. These visual supports will help the students to:
   - Establish and maintain attention.
   - Stay focussed to get complete instructions.
   - Clarify instructions.
   - Perform to completion.
3. *Visual Strategies to Organise the Environment*: Structuring the environment with labelling provides an opportunity for more independence for children with ASD. Certain techniques are:
   - Teach students to recognise the labels and information that already occur naturally in the environment.
   - Label the student's personal spaces and personal belongings.
   - Label where things belong, labelling can show where item belong on a shelf, what is in drawers and where finished work should be put.
   - Labelling the environment name to all activities and label the various activity areas for *e.g.* work area, play area, break area.
4. *Mediating Communication between Environments*: Visual bridge are designed to mediate communication between environments. There are three main goals when implementing this system:

   Goal 1. Mediate communication between home and school or other significant environments.

Goal 2. Stimulate and expand functional language, communication, reading and writing and academic development.

Goal 3. Provide more opportunities for the student to engage in communication and conversation about his experiences.

The method works with children diagnosed as Asperger's ADHD, LD and traumatic brain injury who have problems with communication and are visual learners.

B. Treatment and Education of Autistic and Communication Handicapped Children (TEACCH)

TEACCH founded by Dr. Eric Schopler. TEACCH is more of a philosophy of treatment rather than a specific method. Practitioners of TEACCH make use of several techniques and methods in various combinations depending upon the individual's needs and emerging capabilities.

The curriculum to communication developed by TEACCH emphasises teaching student to communicate more meaning for more purposes in more situations. It also emphasise the use of naturalistic teaching situation with naturalistic consequences, and include procedures for moving teaching into less and less overtly structured settings.

Dimensions of the TEACCH Communication Curriculum

The influence of both behavioural and psycho-linguistic approaches are apparent in TEACCH curriculum. The basis for programming provides a thorough individualised assessment of each child in order to plan an appropriate intervention. The steps are:

1. *Assessment Process*

The purpose of assessment is to identify the child's present communication skills and to point out those deficits that can reasonably be expected to change as a result of some planned intervention. The assessment process includes:

(*a*) First information about the student's current functioning in the fine dimensions of communication such as (1) functions, (2) semantic categories, (3) words, (4) forms, and (5) contexts. This sample is taken by the teacher while observing the student engage in everyday activities at school.

The second step is to interview the parents regarding their observations of their child's communication at home and elsewhere. The interview is structured to elicit the parents observations of their child's skill in each of the five dimensions of communication listed above. The information regarding parents priorities for improving their child's communication is included in the curriculum to help the teacher evaluate and rank possible goals.

2. *Analysis of Communicative Sample*

Analysis of communication sample is important to gather information about student's current skills and tells us 'where to begin' when setting teaching objectives.

3. *Identifying Goals*

Goal selection will be completed after the parent interview. Goals which are given the highest priority in teaching programme would be (*a*) realistic for the student in terms of current skills, (*b*) important in terms of improving the student's ability to communicate in everyday situations or providing some essential survival skills, (*c*) valued by the parents in terms of needs and priorities for the child at home.

4. *Selecting Teaching Objectives*

The process for setting objectives involves two basic principles:

(*i*) Objectives should be chosen which are logical steps toward reaching the student's IEP goals.

(*ii*) Objectives should be chosen which build on the student's existing spontaneous communication skills.

5. *Teaching Strategies*

The activities are designed that the student to learn only one new skill at a time and activities are planned functional for the student, even in structured settings. Environment is engineered to provide naturally occurring opportunities and natural consequences options. Generalisation of skills from school to home and home to school is an important outcome with parents collaboration.

6. *Document of Student Progress*

Establishing criteria for each teaching objective which are tailored to the nature of the objective. Collecting data on a regular basis to document student progress and aids in decision-making about future objectives.

The ultimate aim is to improve students everyday communication skills which is tailored as individual activity and group as well to enhance student's social and communication skills.

C. Picture Exchange Communication System (PECS)

PECS was developed by Andrew S. Bondy and Lori A. Frost. The PECS is used to teach the child to locate a communication partner, present a picture of a desired item, and get the item in exchange for the picture. There are no pre-requisite skills for initiating this system. This social communication exchange is based on child-selected reinforcers. The child spontaneously and intentionally initiates the exchange to request a highly desired item. The exchange is completed when the communication partner gives the highly reinforcing item to the child.

Advantages of the PECS are:

- The exchange is obviously intentional and easy to understand.
- The child is taught to take the initiative—to seek a partner and deliver the message.
- The communication is meaningful and highly reinforcing.

One important positive side effect of this system is large number of children who have developed speech following a year or two of starting the programme. There are six phases of PECS training:

Phase 1: Teaching the First Picture Exchange

Find out what object the child consistently wants, a toy or food item without asking the child 'what do you want'? When preferences emerge and place the desired object on the table and picture card of the object between the child and the object. As child reaches for the object helper guides to pick up the picture (two adults needed, to play the helper and receiver of the picture card). Helper guides the child to release the picture into second adults outstretched hand. As soon as the picture touches adults open hand he receives the object in exchange, with a response "Oh, you want (the object)". The child is not asked what he wants or instructions to pick up the picture. The trainer says nothing until the child has put the picture into an open hand. The above mentioned steps continued more times and gradually physical prompting is dropped.

Phase 2: Increasing Spontaneity and Range

In this phase, the adult gradually moves away from the child and also moves the picture further from the child so he learns to

- get the picture,
- go to the adult to initiate the exchange,
- become more spontaneous,
- child learns to exchange card to different people,
- additional picture cards are added,
- eye contact may increases during these sessions, and
- communication board to designed for the child.

Phase 3: Discrimination of Two or More Pictures

In the third phase, the communication board itself is made more complex. With an object in view, the picture option may be that of two pictures on it. One of the designed object, one of something the child would not be interested in, something irrelevant or neutral. If the child gives the correct picture, gets the desired item; if he gives the other picture, he gets the 'irrelevant' object without no special social reaction. Repeat until child selects correctly on 80 per cent of opportunities.

Phase 4: Building Sentences

A child entering this stage should have a communication system of 12–20 pictures. These picture cards should be arranged in categories. In this phase, the child is taught to request using the phrase "I want ....". By end of Phase 4, child usually has 20–50 pictures in the communication book/board and communicates with a variety of people. He learns to request objects seen or out of sight by using the phrase, "I want ....".

Phase 5: Responding to "What do You Want"?

In this stage the child is taught to respond to the direct question "What do you want"? Whether or not the object is in view to different people in different situation. It requires at least 20 opportunities per day.

Phase 6: Commenting in Response to a Question

By the end of the Phase 5, the child started responding "what do you want"? question. Now the child learns to response to a question "What do you see"? With an "I see ..." card. Objects of minor interest are deliberately chosen to reduce the likelihood of upset/difficult behaviour when it is not handed over. Make sure that 'named' object is not given as a reward as the child might think a request had occurred.

By the end of this phase child should respond to request ("What do you want"?) and naming ("what is this? Or what do you see"?) questions incorporated into daily activities 30–50 pictures in a communication book.

Beyond Phase 6: Introducing Additional Language Concepts

Beyond phase 6, vocabulary, adjectives, verbs, prepositions, language concepts, and sentence structure are expanded to more people and settings. Children typically progress through Phases 1 and 2 within a matter of days. Phase 3 training can take from several days to several months. Phases 4 and 5 are mastered in a few weeks.

When started on PECS as pre-schoolers, speech was acquired by a large percentage of the children who had no form of functional or socially appropriate communication skills.

D. Auditory Integration Training (AIT)

AIT was developed by Guy Berard, a French Otolaryngologist. AIT is based on two assumptions:

- Behaviour is a direct result of how well a person hears.
- The hearing mechanism can be retained. As a result, improved hearing leads to improved behaviour.

Key Points of AIT Programme

1. The minimum age for the listener is 3 years old. There is no upper age limit.
2. The listener should be examined by a health care practitioner prior to start of the sessions.
3. The optional schedule provides for 20 listening sessions lasting for 30 minutes, over a 10-day period. In most cases, the listener has two sessions a day for 10 days. At some AIT clinics, the listening sessions are given for 10 consecutive days; however, it is also acceptable to have a 1-or 2-day break, but only after the first 5 days of listening. The number of sessions and length of them are not subject to change until formal research procedures determine that such changes are beneficial.
4. There are two Berard-approved devices currently available for Berard AIT, the Earducator and the Audiokinetron.
5. Berard AIT can be repeated 6 months after the previous programme. Those with a diagnosis of autism should wait us for 9–12 months before participating in AIT again.
6. Audio tests are typically obtained prior to, at the mid-point, and at the end of the 10 hours of listening.
7. The intensity level (volume) during AIT listening sessions should not exceed an average maximum output of 85 dBA (slow scale) and may be set at much lower intensities depending on the individual's comfort level.

8. Once the AIT programme has been started, headphones should not be used for recreational music and other listening. It is well-documented that use of headphones has reversed the benefits obtained from AIT.

Dr. Berard explains his AIT method and summaries case histories of some of his patients with copies of their hearing tests before and after the treatment, in his book "Hearing Equals Behaviour". Numerous pilot studies of the method shows certain results: a reduction in self-stimulatory behaviour, hyperactivity, anxiety, social withdrawal, distractibility and echolalia, and an increase in attention, comprehension, articulation and auditory memory. It is now known yet how AIT affects a person's behaviours.

E. Alternative and Augmentative Communication (AAC) System

All people need to be able to communicate in every setting. They need not only a consistent and dependable primary communication system, but also back up systems. Those who cannot speak need an alternative system. Those who can speak need an augmentative system to support or augument their speech when it is difficult to understand or when it is limited or not available for use.

There are still many adolescents and adults with autism who have no consistent and effective communication system. Many young children with autism are learning to communicate more effectively that alternative and augmentative communication (AAC) system are more commonly available.

Consideration for Making Decisions

When making decisions about AAC systems and planning instruction to expand communication option for those with autism, consider that—

1. Skill development does not follow the normal or expected sequence. A learner may have low test scores and appear to have very limited potential but have the ability to read and spell.
2. Whatever type of AAC system is selected, it must be introduced in the context of making spontaneous requests.

3. Contrary to earlier belief, basic skills such as attending, eye-contact, motor and verbal limitations, symbol matching, or labelling skills are not pre-requisite for communication training. Rather, these basic skills are learned far more meaningfully in the context of communication training.

Implementation of AAC

(1) *Select a Primary Communication System*

Primary communication system selection depends on the learners spontaneous skills, interests and motor abilities. All alternative systems have some limitations, it could be picture system, written/printed word system, sign system. However, for a learner who is verbal, he must be encouraged to continue speaking and to use gestures, cue card and other backup systems to augment that primary system.

(2) *Design a System*

There are many ways to arrange and display pictures and words for communication purposes. They range from hand-made picture, letter or word boards to extremely high-tech systems with speech output. A system must be updated and adapted as the learner's needs and skills change. If the system does not keep pace with the learner's ever changing needs, it will not be used.

(3) *Select Vocabulary*

Vocabulary for initial picture, word or sign systems is selected for its reinforcing value to the learner. Initial vocabulary needs to allow learners to access/request their most valued objects, food, drink or actions. Additional vocabulary depends on age, interests, and the types of problems the learner is likely to encounter each day in various settings.

Guidelines for Instruction

The initial introduction of a new system or vocabulary occurs in the structured and familiar 1:1 play work, or therapy setting at home or in school. The exact location, session structure, and materials will depend on the vocabulary displayed on the system and the learner's age and ability.

(*a*) *Initiate Instruction*: The power of the system is taught in the context of choice and capitalises on the learner's natural gesture-reaching to grab. As the child reaches to grab, the child's hand is shaped to point to a specific picture/word, shaped to form the sign or assisted to pick up the symbol and place it in the interpreter's hand. The interpreter simultaneously verbalises the learner's intent and delivers the requested item.

(*b*) *Expand Instruction*: Schedule several short, highly structured sessions each day to introduce and integrate new vocabulary into the system. Simultaneously set up or engineer many opportunities to use familiar vocabulary in the context of all natural routines of the day to communicate with more people in more setting.

An ACC specialist and ASD specialist are important resources for solving problems when planning and implementing an ACC system.

V. DEVELOPMENT OF PRAGMATIC SKILLS AND CONVERSATIONAL SKILLS INCLUDING TURN-TAKING AND REPAIR STRATEGIES

Children with ASD are more likely to be successful communications in environment that are designed to encourage and support their efforts. Having a good understanding of a child's current level of communicative competence is the first step in developing an appropriate communication intervention programme for child with autism.

A. Development of Pragmatic Skills

Pragmatics refers to the use of language to express ones intentions and get things done in the world (Gleason, 1985).

This can be broken down into four further areas:

1. Understanding meaning in conversation.
2. Interaction (*e.g.* initiation, facial expression).
3. Structural or linguistic rules.
4. The wider influences upon our communication, such as education, culture and background.

Once the children have worked on all the basic interaction skills then go on to look at more abstract concepts. The suggest tips are:

- Options to increase pragmatic awareness *e.g.* facilitating conversational strategies.
- To work also on semantic area of language.
- Introducing basic skills such as good listening etc.
- To relate activities to talking sessions.
- Developing programme to move from the ability in initial conversation and maintenance.
- Facilitate development and maintenance of friendships.

The Social Use of Language Programme (SULP) was designed by Wendy. Rinaldi assists children with autism to improve pragmatic skills.

B. Expanding the Range of Communicative Functions or Purposes

It is important to teach the child to communicate for a variety of purposes. For a child with autism to develop and expand communication the intervention planned in relation to three primary language functions.

1. ***Behavioural Regulation*:** To develop communicative behavioural regulations, the programme includes:
   - Opportunities to request food or objects.
   - Opportunities to make choices among alternatives.
   - Opportunities to protest actions or to reject objects.
   - Opportunities to request cessation of an activity.
   - Opportunities or needs to request assistance.
2. ***Social Interaction*:** These communicative behaviours used to initiate, respond to maintain or terminate social interaction.

3. ***Joint Activity Routines***: Joint activity routines incorporate familiar, repetitive, communicative interactions, providing an effective language learning strategy for children with autism. It allows the child and adult to engage in meaningful, natural social communicative interactions. An additional positive outcome in using joint activity routines is that they teach the child that he can share experiences with others through communication.

C. Turn-Taking

Conversational turn-taking makes the child to take part in communicative exchanges across several conversational turns as both speaker and listener. He asks contingent questions, allows the communicative partner to complete a conversation turn without interrupting, follows the communicative partner's turn with an appropriate utterance, and allows the communicative partner to take a turn in the conversation. For a child with ASD, who has problem in turn-taking conversation use of visual support strategies enhances the learning.

Turn-taking cards: A visual turn-taking card is a card with 'my turn' printed on it (A graphic symbol can also be used depending on the child's ability to understand various visual representation systems). The turn-taking card is passed back and forth between communication partners to visually represent each conversational partner's turn in the conversation.

D. Conversation Repair and ASD

The child with autism can be taught 'repair strategies' which will assist him successfully repairing breakdowns in expressive communication.

1. *'Repair Strategies' in a Verbal Child*

When conversational breakdown occurs, there is a need for the speaker to possess both linguistic and socio-cognitive skills if a repair is to be achieved. He/she needs to be aware that the listener does not understand something and to be ready to modify utterances. Repair skills involve adequate theory of mind. Because the children with autism have significant language comprehension difficulties many communication breakdowns as listeners may occur. These breakdowns transpire when the child does not understand, or responds inappropriately to verbal information. A communication repair strategy that can be used in these situations is to present the misunderstand information visually, either because the information visually, either because the information is given verbally or he doesn't understand the information, whether verbally or visually presented. Many children with autism can easily be mislabelled as being non-compliant when they do not respond to verbal information. Careful consideration should always be given to the child's ability to comprehend and respond to verbal information (as opposed to visual information) in determining the reason for the breakdown in the communication.

2. *Developing Strategies to Repair Breakdown in Communication for the Non-Verbal Child*

Communication breakdowns can occur for the non-verbal child with autism in both receiving and expressing communicative messages.

(*a*) *Breakdowns in Receiving Communication*: The following strategies can be used to prevent breakdowns, or assist the child in repairing breakdowns in communication when receiving information:

- Secure the child's attention prior to communicating by calling his name, or by physically prompting (for *e.g.* touching shoulders).
- Monitor signs of comprehension (child performs appropriate action or attempts to respond expressively).
- Use simple, short sentences.
- Reduce the amount of auditory information given.
- Give the child time to respond before repeating due to the possibility of delayed auditory processing.
- Use of various visual support strategies to ensure that the child understands the message given.

(*b*) *Breakdowns in Expressive Communication*: Strategies for repairing breakdowns in expressive communication includes—

Persistence teaching the child to repeat his communicative attempt, if the communicative partner does not initially understand. This skill must be taught through the use of highly motivating activities, which will keep the child's interest in pursuing the communicative interaction, even though a breakdown has occurred. After the child communicates an unclear message, the communicative partner can respond with 'I don't understand', or 'tell me again' accompanied by an appropriate gesture. The child should be encouraged to repeat the message, given minimum prompting if necessary.

'Show me': After the child learns to be persistent, he should then learn to respond to 'show me' and then be given an appropriate language model if this is successful.

Example. A child approaches an adult, jumps up and down, vocalises loudly and looks at a specific area of the classroom. The adult verbalises 'show me', points to the area of the classroom indicated by the child, and then leads the child over to that area to encourage them to 'show'.

VI. PRETEND AND ROLE PLAY

Vygotsky (1978) claimed that "in play a child always behaves beyond his average age [because] play contains all developmental tendencies in a condensed form". For the majority of children with autism, it would seen that this 'playfulnes' commonly remains latent; they seem to lack the urge to engage spontaneously in 'playful' behaviour in 'free-play' situations, while structured play contexts with an interested adult can reveal indications of their play potential and clear enjoyment of such activities. There is evidence that pragmatic language skills – the ability to use language in appropriate social contexts, are based upon symbolic skills that children exhibit during play.

Studies into the psychology of children's pretend play have evidenced the importance of role playing and narrative at the heart of socialisation and learning to be part of a culture. Vygotsky (1978) recognised that play enables children to learn cultural tools (such as turn taking, queuing, and conversational skills) through the facilitation of adults and/or peers.

Carol Westby, connected language use in children with the development of their symbolic play skills. What she connected, in her assessment of children, is that children's ability to use language coincides with the emergence of predictable symbolic play schemes. To put it roughly, children doesn't use language fully until they can play in symbolic ways. She proposed that simple stimulus response paradigms (read ABA without symbolic play development), aren't enough to build the symbolic cognitive skills necessary to promote the learner's full language development. Therefore, teaching language use and symbolic play skills should go hand in hand.

Westby play scale seemed to lend itself to teaching theory of mind (TOM) skills at very early ages. Symbolic play and improved social attention skills has preceded acquisition of declarative conversational speech. The acquisition of symbolic play skills has not in itself caused conversational speech to develop, but it has marked a level of social awareness that allowed teaching of declarative conversation to be successful. "In no evaluation has a child's meaningful use of language been above his/her cognitive play level... Unless the child possesses the cognitive pre-requisites for the linguistic structures she/he is learning. She/he will not use them in actual interpersonal situations (Carol Westby, 1980).

Pretend Play Skills

Children with autism need to be taught to pretend play. This type of play is important because it helps develop other skills like imagination, creativity, language and social skills. Pretend play becomes a safe way for children to explore their feelings, ideas and environment. This type of play, will not develop on its own in children with autism. Like many other skills, it must be directly taught.

- Start with individual figures first.
  - Many children with autism are naturally attracted to the many play figures they see on TV. Follow the child's lead when buying play figures.

- Introduce play sets
  - Once the child is familiar with the figures, play sets can be introduced.
- Make play scripts
  - Having a play script made before hand can help keep the pretend play flowing.
- Monitor strange behaviour
  - Often children will become excited while playing and story can increase. Redirect this type of behaviour.

Example: Tea Party

(Tea parties helps to expand imagination and pretending skills in the following progression).

- *Initial Target*: Learner will participate in a real tea party with real food and drinks.
- *Second Target*: Learner will participate in a tea party with realistic toy food.
- *Third Target*: Learner will participate in a tea party with imaginary food.
- *Fourth Target*: Learners will offer food and beverages to stuffed animals and dolls/action figures who participate in the tea party.
- *Final Target*: Learner will offer food and beverages to typical peer who participate in the tea party.

Role-Play

Most children with autism do not develop spontaneous symbolic play, yet when prompted to play, those that have symbolic capacity in their language may begin to use symbolic acts and play materials.

The role-play of children with autism is often stereotypical and tends not to involve attributing a mental state to inanimate objects (for example, 'my Dolly is hungry') when entering into role-play, a child follows and improvises upon the flexible narrative of another-often the words are not scripted and the child must take on some of the surface characteristics to signify that the role has been taken;

these characteristics are incorporated into the child's own understanding of the world. It follows, that the relative lack of role play in children with autism contributes to their later difficulty in understanding the minds of others.

Enabling Pretence in Children with Autism

Research has shown that it is possible to shape the emergence of pretend play in children with autism, through systematically rewarding desired symbolic play acts *e.g.* role playing – pretending to cook dinner. It appears that there is a positive relationship between language skills and levels of prompted pretend play in children with autism. In order for children with autism to develop symbolic play, it appears necessary to prompt them in same way. Using a clear structure may reduce the need for prompting time.

The thought process responsible for creative representations in symbolic pretend play are similar to those involved in social understanding, the social use of language and some aspects of semantic language that require highly fluid understanding of changing meaning.

Summary

Each person with an ASD has different communication skills. Some people may have relatively good verbal skills, others man does not speak at all or have limited ability or interest in communicating and interacting with others. About 40% of children with ASDs do not talk at all. The communication difficulties related to autism can be much more complicated and subtle-they can be related to the social uses of language and in using non-verbal language to communicate as well.

No one treatment method has been found to successfully improve communication in all individuals with ASD. A number of communication focused interventions are commonly used with children with ASD. These may be used in isolation or integrated into a more comprehensive programme. A holistic communication programme focuses on developing different means for communication selection of particular communication is based upon the child's current level of communicative competence.

5

Sensory Motor and Self-Help Skill Training

I. MOTOR EXECUTIVE DYSFUNCTION IN ASD

Executive functions are important for successful adaptation and performance in red life situations. They allow people to initiate and complete tasks and to preserve in the face of challenges. Because, the environment can be unpredictable, executive functions are vital to human ability to recognise the significance of unexpected situations and to make alternative plans quickly when unusual events arise and interfere with normal routines. Executive functions also enable people to inhibit inappropriate behaviours. Executive functions also enable people to inhibit inappropriate behaviours. Executive functions are an important component of the ability to fit in socially.

Definition

The term executive function describes a set of cognitive abilities that control and regulate other abilities and behaviours. Executive functions are necessary for good oriented behaviour. They include the ability to initiate and stop actions, to monitor and change behaviour as needed, and to plan future behaviour when faced with novel tasks and situations. Executive functions allow us to anticipate outcomes and adapt to changing situations. The ability to form concepts and think abstractly are often considered components of executive function.

Executive Dysfunction in Autism

Over the past twenty years several executive functions have been studies in autism. The diagnosis of this problem has only been available in the last 7-10 year as advanced technologies allowed new observations of brain function.

The presence of executive function deficit in ASD has been the subject of several investigations, the nature of the executive function problems in ASD are less established. For example, several questions remain; the profile of executive function deficits, specificity of executive function deficit to ASD, and presence across the life span remain to be established. Ozonoff and colleagues provide a comprehensive review of executive function research in ASD and suggest that when evaluating components of executive function in ASD, a consistent pattern of abilities and disabilities appear. Generally, the literature suggests that sustained attention and response inhibition are two components of executive function that are relatively preserved in ASD. In contrast, set shifting/ flexibility and planning are commonly found deficits. Deficits in other executive functions are more mixed, particularly in the area of working memory.

Happe and colleagues investigated executive function in males age 8-16 years with ASD or ADHD and typically developing children. The study utilised multiple measures of skills in three executive function domains, namely response selection, flexibility and planning/ working memory. Results indicated the clinical groups performed below typically developing children on all but one variable measuring response selection. Additionally, the ADHD patients exhibited greater impairments than the ASD. The results also found age related improvements in executive function in children with ASD, but not ADHD. These findings suggest that observed problems in executive function in ASD may relate to delayed brain maturation in which the frontal cortices are the last to achieve full functionality, rather than an autism-specific executive function deficit.

Sensory Motor Deficits in Autism

The majority of infants with autism attain basic motor milestones essentially 'on time', numerous studies also provide evidence that motor problems may sometimes be quiet significant. Specific deficits have been reported, including in motor imitation, balance, coordination, finger-to-thumb opposition, muscle tone, postural stability, motor control, motor stereotypes, sensory and arousal modulation, and speech articulation. Unusual sensory-perceptual reactions appear to be manifest in some children with autism as early as first year of life.

Table 5.1: Shared Symptom Domains and Associated Psycho-social Interventions in ASD

Symptom Domain	*Description of Deficit*	*ASD Treatments*
Motor Skills	*ADHD and ASD*: Evidence strongest for ! deficits in higher level, motor coordination deficits in both disorders.	*Sensory integration thera-pies*: Limited empirical support. *Physical therapy*: No treatment studies in ASD
Executive Functions	*ADHD*: Consistent findings of deficits in inattention, inhibition, and working memory.	*Organisational skills/cognitive remediation*: No published treatment studies in ASD
	ASD: Some support for deficits in set-shifting and flexibility but not consistent.	*Computerised cognitive training interventions*: No published treatment studies in ASD
		ABA, PBS: RCTs show improvements in variety of disruptive behaviours including impulsivity, inattention

Conclusion. The study of the overlap in symptom domains of motor coordination, executive function in ASD is relatively recent. Data on motor coordination difficulties suggests the presence of motor dysfunction across many developmental disorders, including ASD. These findings may relate to the relative vulnerability of the motor system to developmental insult. Additional research on this symptom domain may have implications for motor skills as a shared endophenotype across disorders. The failure to find ASD specific deficits in studies utilising controls for delay or disability may provide support to the intriguing, yet controversial concept of DAMP (deficit in attention, motor control and perception), which proposes a syndrome characterised by deficits in motor-coordination, inattentive symptom and deficit in visual-perceptual abilities, and which has high co-occurrence in ASDs. Research continues to evaluate the presence and specificity of executive function deficits in ASDs. Psycho-social treatments for behavioural deregulation related to executive function have strong empirical support and primarily include behavioural interventions based in operant conditioning theory. Promising psycho-social treatments for other executive function domains such as attention, and organisational/planning skills may provide interesting avenues for application in ASD.

II. SENSORY INTEGRATION THERAPY (SIT)

To function and participate in the world that surrounds us, we need to use our senses. Senses provide individuals with unique experiences and allow us to interact and be involved with the rest of society. They help us to understand the environment around us and respond within it. They play a significant role in determining what actions we take in a particular situation.

A. Sensory Process

In order to receive information present in the environment human being is provided with sense organs. The process of receiving information in the form of its respective force and transmitting the same to the central nervous system in the form of electrical transmission is the sensory process. We are all familiar with the five basic sensory systems. Sight (visual), ear (auditory), nose (olfactory), tongue (gustatory), skin (tactile), known as external senses. The internal senses are:

Sl. No.	*Organ*	*Function*	*System*
1.	Muscle spindle	Awareness of body movements	Proprioceptive system
2.	Organ of balance	Noticing every movement and position of head in relation to gravity	Vestibular system
3.	Muscle joint		Kinaesthetic system
4.	Inner organs	Gives information on our well-being	Vicera system

B. Sensory Integration Theory

Dr. A. Jean Ayres, an occupational therapist and psychologist, was the first researcher, clinician developed the concept of sensory integration. The sensory integration theory proposes that sensory integration is a neurobiological process that organises sensation from one's own body and from the environment and makes it possible to use the body effectively within the environment. The spatial and temporal aspects of inputs from different sensory modalities are interpreted, associated and unified. Sensory integration is information processing, praxis (motor planning) and perception are both end products of sensory integration.

Ayres sensory integration includes the theory, assessment, patterns of sensory integration, and praxis dysfunction and intervention concepts, principles and techniques articulated by Ayres and applied by therapist trained in this approach worldwide. Ayres developed IT standardised tests and many non-standardised observation that contributed to the identification and understanding of the multiple patterns of sensory integration dysfunction.

Common Patterns of Sensory Integration Dysfunctions

This includes visual perception deficits; visual motor deficits; visual construction and praxis deficits (visuo dyspraxia); factile-discrimination deficit; vestibular processing deficits; proprioceptive processing deficits and poor body scheme; bilateral integration and sequencing deficits including poor postural control (bilateral integration and sequencing); somatosensory-based dyspraxia, language-based dyspraxia, sensory sensitivities especially tactile defensiveness and gravitational insecurity.

Patterns of sensory integration dysfunction that include motor in coordination, fine and gross motor delays, deficits in balance, poor praxis are often included in the diagnostic category of developmental coordination disorder. Patterns of sensory integration dysfunction that include unusual over, under or fluctuating responses to sensation may be included in deficits such as sensory processing disorder or regulatory disorder.

C. Sensory Integration Challenges in ASD

Sensory impairment, or differences in the processing sensory information, affects many children with ASD. Sensory input may be heightened (hyper), reduced (hype) or inconsistent and this can have far reaching consequences for a child's intellectual, social, emotional and motor development.

Sensory problems may be related to difficulties with arousal levels. The state of arousal of children with ASD is often too high or too low. This may result in a variety of difficulties for the child, including problems with impulse control, problems with focussing and maintaining attention, sleeping difficulties, etc.

Sensory problems may affect a child's ability to control or 'filter' incoming sensory information from their surroundings. As a result the child may not be able to organise or make use of the sensory input received. They may be unable to tune out irrelevant stimuli, be hypersensitive or hypersensitive to certain stimuli, or have fluctuating perceptual skills.

An inability to tune out irrelevant sensory information may have many consequences, for existence – it may make it difficult for a child to hear a single voice above other sounds or to see a person or object as something distinct from their surroundings. This may explain why a child with ASD prefers things to remain consistent or unchanged. It may also result in sensory overload which is probably not a pleasant experience. Children may use actions and behaviours to reduce this affect, such as tuning out, using peripheral vision or focussing intently on something to block out other sensory input.

Hypersensitivity may result in a range of behaviours in response to stimuli as stimuli may be experienced as painful or pleasurable. Children with hypersensitivities may use behaviours or actions to reduce, block out or to create pleasing sensory experiences.

Hyposensitivity may result in delayed, limited or no response to stimuli. Hyposensitive children may use activities or self-stimulating behaviours to excite or arouse their nervous system. Fluctuating sensory performance will probably lead to inconsistent behaviours and functioning by a child.

Sensory issues do not automatically have negative consequences – a heightened auditory sense may give a person a good ear for music, heightened visual skills may help in artistic or scientific pursuits, etc.

D. Sensory Integration Therapy

Sensory integration therapy involves the gentle exposure to various sensory stimuli. The aim of this therapy is to strengthen, balance, and develop the central nervous systems processing of sensory stimuli. Delacato (1974), who introduced the concept of sensory integration therapy, focussed the therapy on the five core sensory systems—vision, taste, smell, auditory and tactility. Today, occupational therapists continue to focus on these areas, as well as incorporating the vestibular and proprioception system, when creating and planning a schedule of activities for an individual. Techniques usually focus on stimulating vestibular sense (*i.e.* motion, balance), the tactile sense (*i.e.* touch), and on proprioception (*e.g.* joints, ligaments), in order to make them less or more sensitive and to help a child to recognise sensory information.

Organisation of senses. The tactile, vestibular, and proprioceptive systems begin to function very early in life, even before birth. These basic senses are closely connected to each other systems of the brain as development proceeds. The interplay among the various senses is complex, and is necessary in order for a person to interpret a situation accurately and make an appropriate response. It is this organisation of the senses for use that is termed sensory integration.

Motor planning (praxis). Praxis in an end product of sensory integration. Motor planning (praxis) is an important ability that depends on efficient sensory integration. Motor planning involves having an idea about what to do, planning an action, and finally executing the action. The tactile, proprioceptive, and vestibular senses are particularly important in providing knowledge about how the body moves and how it can be used to act on the environment. Motor planning involves conscious attention to the task, while relying on stored information regarding unconscious body sensation. Because many sensory process takes place within the nervous system at unconscious level, we are not usually aware of them.

Sensory integration therapy usually given by specially trained occupational therapists who observe the child carefully to gain a clear understanding of his particular sensitivities. Experts and researchers disagree about whether these kinds of therapies really work or if they are scientifically valid. Some people have found that when the sensory needs of autism are met, learning is more focussed, progress is better and people are better able to cope with day-to-day situations. Addressing sensory issues may be a very long process. In addition, physical therapy and exercise can be helpful for people with autism who have limited gross and fine motor skills.

E. Assessment and Intervention

1. Identifying children with SI dysfunction
2. Standardised assessment
   - Informal clinical observation
   - Parent interview
   - Observation at home or in school especially beneficial for autistic population
3. What happens in treatment?
   - Generally a positive experience
   - Activities designed to be appropriate at child's developmental level
   - Compelling but not overwhelming challenge in order to promote growth and exploration
   - Self-motivation of child is important, not highly structured treatment
   - Children with low arousal – intense, frequently changing sensations
   - Children with high arousal – calming activities, slow, rhythmic sensations
   - Set-up environment to encourage motor planning, variety of changing equipment
   - Safety to experiment with movement
   - Parent consultation and education is pertinent. In treatment and intervention constantly creating opportunities for adaptive responses to get the feedback and to lead for further learning.
4. Creating of a sensory diet and accommodations with parents and case workers
5. Evaluation

Upon completion of the sensory integration treatment the child show success in daily activities, less frustration, less avoidance of task or interactions less need for assistance. Also better organisation of behaviour, increased adaptability, improved motor skills and greater confidence.

III. LIFE SPAN SKILL MANAGEMENT

Traditional occupational therapy often is provided to promote development of self-care skills (*e.g.* dressing, manipulating fasteners, using utensils, personal hygiene) and academic skills (*e.g.* waiting, fine motor). Occupational therapist also may assist in prompting development of play skills modifying classroom materials and routines to improve attention and organisation, and providing prevocational training. However, research regarding the efficacy of occupational therapy in ASD is lacking. Sensory Integration (SI) therapy often is used alone as part of a broader programme of occupational therapy for children with ASDs.

Occupational Therapy Intervention for Children with Autism

The goal of occupational therapy interventions is to enable individuals to participate in everyday occupations. This may be achieved through a range of therapy approaches modification of tasks and/or the environment to match individuals abilities, developing skills such as posture and coordination, or development of daily routines to facilitate adaptive behaviours. There is a need for more research and evidence to support best approaches to enhancing the participation of children with autism in the occupation of daily life. The majority of occupational therapist (82%) currently addressing in praxis, self-regulation oral motor/ feeding and sensory integration.

Occupational therapy is a health profession that is directed toward enabling people to participate in daily occupations, including care of oneself, contributing to society (*e.g.* paid and unpaid work, school and enjoying life (*e.g.* hobbies, sports). Occupational therapy evaluation is designed to gain an understanding of the individual's abilities and difficulties in performing daily occupations; it looks at the child's development in a number of domains including motor, perceptual, communication and interaction skills, habits and routines.

Occupational Therapist's Role in Skills Training

The occupational therapy focus to make contributions in enabling people to acquire and re-acquire skills and to improve the quality of life. In occupations therapy, the focus is on task analysis, breaking down a task into meaningful steps, teaching those steps to the key people in the environment and structuring task and/or environment to support successful completion.

Adaptable Teaching Techniques

In occupational therapy, a skill is defined as a performance component which evolves with practice. Performance is the process or manner of functioning, which incorporates what a person does and how it is done. Performance is the outward expression of skills. Aspects of cognition are essential to the development of performance. Associated skills are restricted if there are problems in cognition.

The contribution of occupational therapy to life and skills training earlier built on by Mosey and Kielhofner, Ayre's work, which later became the 'sensory integration theory' and Llorens, emphasised on activities, tasks and interpersonal interactions to reinstate skills.

Task Oriented Activities

Traditionally, in occupational therapy, task oriented activities are associated with the concept of doing, be it a practical, functional or creative activity. A task is a constituent past of an activity. It is through the precise analysis of activities broken down into tasks that the learning process in occupational therapy is often facilitated.

Four practice models and approaches:

1. The model of human occupation (Kielhofner, 1985)
2. Cognitive disabilities model (Allen, 1982)
3. Mosey's adaptive skills approach (1970)
4. Model of adaptation through occupation (Reed and Sanderson, 1984)

Each model has its own perspective on how to develop and harness certain skills. It is suggested that each model has its contribution to make in facilitating the acquisition or reestablishment of skills, depending on the individual's circumstances. A pragmatic and holistic approach in their use is therefore advised independent life and community participation skills is important and some model programme provide programming throughout childhood and adulthood. When child with ASDs move beyond preschool and early elementary programmes, educational interventions continues, in adolescence, the term 'transition' is used to describe the movement from child-centred activities to adult oriented activities. The emphasis may shift from academic to vocational services from remediating deficits to fostering abilities. Comprehensive transition planning involves the student, parents, teachers, the medical home, and representatives from all concerned community agencies. Depending on the individual's cognitive level, social skills, health condition, work habits, and behavioural challenges, preparation for competitive, supported or sheltered employment is targetted. Regardless of the type of employment, attention to skill development should never stop. Skills necessary for independent living should be taught to the degree possible given the abilities of the person. Available studies are plagued by methodological limitations, but proponents of sensory integration note that higher quality SI research is forthcoming. 'Sensory' activities may be helpful as part of an overall programme that uses desired sensory experiences to calm the ASDs, reinforce a desired behaviour, or help with transition between activities.

Many of the specific challenges of people with autism necessitate careful planning for the transition into adulthood and for transitions of all types throughout the life span.

IV. ALTERNATE THERAPIES

Sensory integration therapy includes a variety of different interventions, some that occur in a natural setting, others that are less natural but necessary.

A. Berard Auditory Integration Therapy (AIT)

Guy Berard, a French Otolaryngologist developed auditory integration training (AIT) and special AIT devices – Audiokinetron, and the Earducator. According to Berard, the auditory dysfunction is due to biological causes and the processing problems may occur if a person hears some frequencies better than the others and develops 'auditory peaks' (frequencies to which a person is hypersensitive).

AIT is based on two assumptions:

1. Behaviour is a direct result of how well a person hears.
2. The hearing mechanism can be retained. As a result, improved hearing leads to improved behaviour.

B. Irlen Lense System

Helen Irlen, a former school psychologist and current Assistant Professor of Adult Learning Disabilities at California, estimates that almost 50 per cent of people with autism have scotopic sensitivity, or unusual sensitivity to lights, glare, patterns, colours and contrasts. Drawing on federal research from the early 1980s, Irlen developed what are now known as Irlen Lenses to filter out colours of the infrared spectrum that interfere with visual perception in person on the autism spectrum.

Scotopic sensitivity is triggered by one or more components of light, such as the source of the light (*e.g.* fluorescent lighting, sun) luminance (*e.g.* reflection, glare), intensity (*i.e.* brightness), wave length (*i.e.* colour), and/or colour contrast. People with scotopic sensitivity/Irlen syndrome experience 'perceptual stress' which can lead to a variety of perceptual distortions when reading/or viewing the environment. As a result, the person may experience:

- *Light Sensitivity*: Bothered by brightness, glare, types of lightening.
- *Inefficient Reading*: Letters on page move, dance, vibrate, jiggle.
- *Inadequate Background Accommodations*: Difficulty with high contrast.
- *Restricted Span of Recognition*: Tunnel vision or difficulty reading groups of letters.
- *Lack of Sustained Attention*. Difficulty maintaining attention.

The Irlen lense system developed by Irlen, was designed to treat scotopic sensitivity/Irlen syndrome. She has developed two methods to treat scotopic sensitivity:

1. The use of coloured transparencies or overlays to improve reading; and
2. Tinted glasses to improve one's visual perception of his/her environment.

There is growing evidence, based on both research and personal reports, that many autistic individuals see their world in a maladaptive, dysfunctional manner. Additionally there are many visual problems which are often associated with autism, such as hand-flapping and finger-flicking.

Recently there have appeared reports about changes people with autism experience while using coloured lenses that give another evidence that there are some visual-perceptual abnormalities in autism. This type of visual perceptual deficits associated with autism is unique, and the distortions are varied, unpredictable and constantly changing.

Quite a few autistic individual's have reported positive changes in their visual hypersensitivity brought by the tinted filters. The positive changes are perception with depth instead of two dimensional world, no fragmentation of visual information, improvement in eye contact, the ability to use several channels at the same time (*e.g.* to see and to hear), reduced sensitivity to auditory stimuli, increased ability to understand language, and better small and gross motor coordination.

The Irlen method is not a 'cure' for autism but rather one of the tools or compensatory strategies to reduce hypersensitivities and distortions of visual perception.

C. Vision Therapy

A variety of visual therapies such as—

- *Oculomotor Exercises*: Performing eye movement exercises to reorganise and normalise the visual system.
- *Irlen Lenses*: Wearing ambient (prison) lenses have been used with children with autism in attempts to improve visual processing or visual-spatial perception. There are no empirical studies regarding the efficacy of the use of Irlen lenses or occulomotor therapies specifically in children with autism. Prism lenses are purported to

produce more stable visual perception and improved behaviour or performance by shifting the field of vision through an angular displacement of 1 to 5 degrees (base up or base down). Only one study investigated the use of prism lenses in children with autism, almost half of whom also had strabismus. Results indicated some short-term positive behavioural effects with less improvement at later follow up.

D. Hippotherapy

The term hippotherapy refers to a therapeutic horseback riding programme. Specially trained physical and occupational therapists use this method of treating children with special needs to improve circulation and respiration and to help them develop strength, coordination, balance, self-confidence and patience.

Hippotherapy focusses on organising the inner and outer senses. However, with this unique modality, the child rides on the back of a horse. A therapist acquainted with hippotherapy and a specially trained horse conduct hippotherapy session. The child heightens her awareness by developing her vestibular and proprioceptive senses, which she accomplishes through using her trunk muscles to maintain balance on the horse. Additionally, the child benefits psychologically by learning how to communicate with and develop a relationship with the horse. It is a session with fun. Generally therapists can adapt hippotherapy to assist children across the autism spectrum.

E. Pressure Techniques

(*i*) *The Wilbarger Protocol*: Some children have a tendency to respond to certain harmless sensations as if they were dangerous or painful. This is called sensory defensiveness (SD). The child with SD may misperceive the world as dangerous, alarming or at the very least irritating. The protocol uses frequent application of firm/deep pressure touch input to various parts of the body. This is followed by gentle joint compression.

(*ii*) *Weighted Vest*: The concept of the weighted vest is based on the technique of deep pressure. Deep pressure is used to assist the child to self-calm and relax so that sensory stimulus can be processed. The use of weighted vest is thought to provide the child with unconscious information from the muscles and joints. Children who are easily distracted, hyperactive and lacking in concentration are said to respond positively to the additional weight arrest provides.

(*iii*) *Weighted Blanket*: The weighted blanket is behaved by some to have a similar calming effect to other pressure techniques. Due to the fact that weighted blankets can cover more of the body there have been some safety concerns associated with the use of weighted blankets for children.

(*iv*) *Squeeze Machine*: The 'squeeze machine' or 'Hug Box' was developed by Temple Grandin. It is made of two padded side-boards which are hinged near the bottom to form a V-shape. The user lies down or squats inside the V. By using a lever, the user engages an air cylinder, which pushes the side-boards together. This action provides the deep pressure stimulation evenly across the lateral parts of the body, which some persons with ASD crave. Some persons prefer long squeeze while others prefer a short one. The machine was designed in such a way that the child could control the amount and duration of the pressure. It helps in tolerating touch and which appears to have a calming effect.

F. Perceptual-Motor Development Therapy

Kephart was one of the first researcher to incorporate neurological networks in his theory of development (i.e., behaviour is ultimately defined by a "neurological process"). He believes that development of most behaviours arises from a hierarchy of motor achievement.

The central care of Kephart's theory is that motoric responses to a child's environment is the central care to all behaviour. Motor activity = behaviour is not an over exaggeration of his ideas, he stated it as a perceptual motor match. Kephart believed that all perceptual development rises from a hierarchy of motor skills, his hierarch includes

(*a*) movement control,

(*b*) systematic exploration,
(*c*) perception,
(*d*) intersensory integration,
(*e*) concept formation.

In order to achieve each stage of hierarchy, Kephart proposed four bases of motor learning:

1. *Posture*: A basic movement pattern that allows the child to wage the war against gravity
   (*i*) Serves as a point of reference.
   (*ii*) Sefely function while learning more complicated motor tasks.
2. *Laterality*: Recognition of the two symmetrical halves of the body.
   (*i*) The ability to detect the two different sides, not name them.
   (*ii*) Important for keeping balance as more difficult motor tasks are attempted.
3. *Directionality*: Translation of laterality cues to objects in free space.
   (*i*) Relative position of two objects is understood.
   (*ii*) Requires fairly developed age and hand movement.
4. *Body image*: Knowledge of different body parts in reference to the child's midline as well as to on another.
   (*i*) Relationship to other objects in space is also a confinement.

After achieving the "four bases" the child is able to move about with some purpose. To learn effectively from the environment, the child must learn four basic movement patterns. He developed a battery Purdue's perceptual-motor survey to evaluate child's perceptual-motor development components of perceptual-motor efficiency cover a broad spectrum of perceptual abilities: (*a*) postural and loco-motor awareness, (*b*) auditory perception and antianchrory spatial awareness, (*c*) visual perception and visual spatial awareness, (*d*) kinesthetic perception, (*e*) factile perception, (*f*) body awareness, and (*g*) laterality and directionality. Cognitive development also involves the introduction and learning of basic academic concepts. Educators are now recognizing that important perceptual motor skills and fundamental academic concepts can be effectively delt with in a movement education programme and this showed a good improvement in children with ASD.

Summary

Many children with autism experience sensory and motor difficulties at point in their development. These include order or over-reactions to basic sensations and perceptions, movement and formation from muscles and joints. The sensory challenges in ASDs are more complex and confusion occurs in the sensory channel. Most person with ASDs, regardless at which point they many fall alongwith the continuum of intellectual and communication abilities, have difficulty with attention and executive functions of self-monitored organizational skills.

The use of intensive sensor motor therapy activities far very significantly impaired persons with autism who fail to relate or have little interest in their environment, and who do not communicate verbally, is strongly recommended. This emphasis on almost continuous SI activities and will be the basis for the child to eventually organize his world and to be able to respond day-to-day's activities, vocational activities, and other activities which can promote his communication and learning. Remember that teaching skills (SI) only in therapy sessions is madequate—These techniques and supports must be integrated into their everyday lives. Teaching and supporting independent life skills is important for facilitating positive social lives for people with ASDs.

Bibliography

Albin, R.W. and R.H. Horner (1988): Generalization with precision. In Generalization and Maintenance: Life-style changes in applied settings, edited by R.H. Horner, G. Dunlap, and R.L. Koegel, 99-120. Baltimore: Paul H. Brookers.

Anderson, J. (1998): Sensory Motor Issues in Autism. San Antoniono, TX: Therapy Skill Builders.

Attwood, A.J. (1993): Movement disorders and autism: a rationale for the use of facilitated communication and an alternative model for training staff and students.

Ayres, J.A. (1979): Sensory Integration and the child, Los Angeles: Western psychological services.

Baron-Cohen, S. (1988): Social and Pragmatic deficits in autism: cognitive or affective? Journal of Autism and Developmental Disorders 18: 379-402.

Beisler, J.M., & Tsai, L.Y. (1983): A pragmatic approach to increase language skills in young autistic children. Journal of Autism and Developmental Disorder, 13, 287-303.

Berard. G. (1993): Hearing Equals Behaviour, New Canaan, Connecticut: Keats Publishing.

Bondy, A.S., and L.A. Frost (1994): The Picture Exchange System: Focus on Autism behaviour.

Coleman, M. (1990): Autism : Non-drug biological treatments. In Diagnosis and treatment of autism, edited by C. Gillman, New York: Plenum Press.

Earr, E.G. (1985): Behavioural approaches to language and communication. In E. Schopler & G.B. Mesibov (Eds), communication problems in autism (pp. 37-57) New York: Plenum.

Frith, U. (1989): Autism: Explaining the enigma. Oxford, England: Black Well.

Grandin. T. (1990): 'Sensory problem in autism' paper presented at the 1990 Arrival conference of the Autism Society of America, Buena Park, California, 1990.

Handen, B.L. (1993): Pharmacotherapy in mental retardation and autism. School Psychology Review 22(2): 162-183.

Harty, J.R. (1990): Pharmacotherapy in Infantile autism. Focus on Autistic Behaviour 5:2.

Hodgdon, Linda, A. (1995): Visual Strategies to Enhance communication in children with Autism, Quirk Robert Publishing, Michigan.

Horner, R.H. (1994): Facilitated communication keeping it practical. Journal of the Association for persons with severe Handicaps (JASH) 19(3): 185-186.

Kierman, C. (1983): The use of non-vocal communication techniques with autistic individuals. Journal of child psychology and psychiatry 24, 339-375.

Klinger, L.G., and G. Dawson (1992): Facilitating easily social & communicative development in children with autism.

Kranowitz, C. (1998): The out of sync child: Recognizing and coping with Sensory Integration Dysfunction. New York; Skylight Press.

Linda R. Watson, Catherine Lord, Bruce Schaffer, Eric Schopler: Teaching Spontaneous communication to Autistic and Developmentally Handicapped Children.

Lovaas, O.I. (1977): The autistic child, New York: irrigation.

Lovaas, O.I. Simmons, J.Q. Koegel, R.L. & Stevens-Long, J. (1973): Some generalization and follow-up measures on autistic children in behaviour therapy. Journal of Applied Behaviour Analysis, 6, 131-166.

Maurice, C. (1997): Behavioural Intervention for children with Autism, pro-ed Texas, US.

Menyak, P. & Quill, K. (1985): Semantic problems in autistic children. In E. Schopler & G. Mesibov (Eds), communication problems in autism (pp. 127-145), New York: Plenum.

Prizant, B. (1983): Language and communication in autism: Toward an understanding of the "Whole" of it. Journal of Speech & Hearing Disorders, 48, 296-307.

Prizant, B.M. (1982): Gestalt language and gestalt processing in autism. Topics in Language Disorder, 3, 16-23.

Quil, K. (1991): Methods to Enhance student learning communication and self control. Autism society of America conference proceedings Indianapolis, In: ASD.

Rimland, B. (1990): 'Sound Sensitivity in autism' Autism Research Review International 4, 1 and 6.

Rimland, B., and S. Edelson (1994): The effects of auditory integration training on autism American Journal of Speech-Language Pathologists 5(5): 16-24.

Siegal, B. (1996): The world of the Autistic child: Understanding and treating Autistic Spectrum Disorder. New York: Oxford University Press.

Sunderberg, M. and Partington, J.W. (1995): Teaching Language to children with Autism and other Developmental disabilities, Behaviour Analysis. Inc. CA.

Tirosh, E. and Canby, J. (1993): Autism with Hyperlexia: A distinct syndrome?' American Journal of Mental Retardation.

Ungerer, J.A. & Sigman, M. (1981): Symbolic play and language comprehension in autistic children. Journal of the American Academy of child psychiatry. 20, 318-337.

Wing, L. and Attwood, A. (1987): 'Syndromes of autism and a typical development.' In D. Cohen and A. Donnellan (eds.) Handbook of Autism and pervasive developmental disorders. New York: John Miley & Sons.

